Joggin' Your Noggin

More Challenging Word Activities for Seniors

Volume Four

Mary Randolph, M.S., CCC
Speech-Language Pathologist

ISBN:1503154211
ISBN-13:9781503154216

Copyright © 2015 Mary Randolph

All rights reserved.

DEDICATION

To our dear mother, Helen, whose struggle with Alzheimer's disease inspired the development of the "Joggin' Your Noggin" series of books, puzzles and games. Mom never lost her wonderful ability to enjoy and appreciate the moment, despite challenges resulting from her progressive, debilitating illness. Helen passed away peacefully at the end of 2013. Her lessons taught us to face every obstacle with courage and conviction; to look for the positive in people and situations; to respect diversity; to be thankful for blessings; to strive to make a difference; and to recognize the value of every new day.

INTRODUCTION

This latest in the "Joggin' Your Noggin" series once again affords hours of stimulating fun to people faced with diminishing mental ability. Though originally intended for individuals suffering from dementia, the books also receive positive reviews from many others, including people suffering from stroke, traumatic brain injury or exposure to Agent Orange.

The entertaining and challenging word activities can be completed individually, with a family member/caregiver, or in a group. A retired speech-language pathologist, the author has over twenty years' experience helping adults and children develop language and communication skills. These "games" might be considered a type of calisthenics for the brain, great exercise for memory and word recall. This edition focuses on common word associations, synonyms, antonyms, compound words and categories. For example, a phrase like "Bread and _____" triggers the word "butter." In the case of famous people, the name "Abbot" evokes the associated name "Costello." Given several words, "cow, sheep, zebra, duck," the word "zebra" does not fit as it is not a farm animal. Synonyms include two words with the same meaning, and antonyms are two words with opposite meanings. Compound words are comprised of two smaller words, such as "bookmark." Answers are provided on the page following each "game" for easy accessibility. **Please note** that only one, or a small sample, of many possible correct answers is provided.

The Appendix contains reproducible "Bingo" boards that facilitate an interactive group activity based on items in the book. Simple directions are included.

TABLE OF CONTENTS

Game #	Title	Page #
1	Exclusions	1-10
2	Word Pairs--Objects	11-22
3	Rhyming Words	23-30
4	Opposites	31-42
5	Synonyms	43-54
6	Cartoon Characters	55-58
7	Famous Duo's	59-62
8	Capitals & Places	63-74
9	Categories	75-98
10	Animal Young	99-102
11	Animal Homes	103-106
12	Animal Parts	107-110
13	Animal Sounds	111-114
14	"Name Something…"	115-122
15	"Name a Word that Describes…"	123-130
16	Compound Words	131-142
Appendix	"Bingo" Boards	143-179

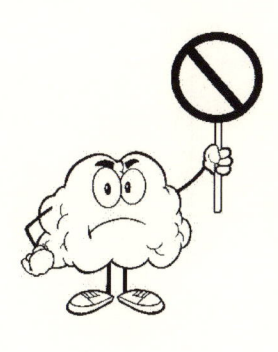

NAME THE ONE THAT DOES NOT BELONG

1. flute, saxophone, trumpet, drum

2. apple, lime, grapefruit, orange

3. bed, dresser, toaster, lamp

4. robin, ant, flea, beetle

5. tongs, knife, toothbrush, spatula

6. bear, hawk, cat, rabbit

7. ladle, knife, ax, saw

8. Toyota, Ford, Chrysler, Buick

9. elm, oak, daffodil, maple

10. cinnamon, pepper, nuts, sage

ANSWERS TO: NAME THE ONE THAT DOES NOT BELONG

1. Drum is not a wind instrument.

2. Apple is not a citrus fruit.

3. Toaster is not bedroom furniture.

4. Robin is not an insect.

5. Toothbrush is not a kitchen utensil.

6. Hawk is not a four-legged, furry animal.

7. Ladle is not a cutting tool.

8. Toyota is not an American car.

9. Daffodil is not a tree.

10. Nuts are not a spice.

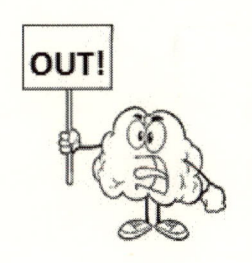

NAME THE ONE THAT DOES NOT BELONG

1. tuna, swordfish, eel, elk
2. terrier, collie, calico, dachshund
3. plaid, striped, cooked, paisley
4. watch, clock, thermometer, stopwatch
5. blonde, brunette, redhead, freckled
6. sled, bulldozer, backhoe, plow
7. revolver, pistol, slingshot, rifle
8. tibia, thumb, pointer, pinkie
9. wheat, barley, oats, acorns
10. week, month, appointment, year

ANSWERS TO: NAME THE ONE THAT DOES NOT BELONG

1. Elk is not a fish.

2. Calico is not a dog.

3. Cooked is not a fabric design.

4. Thermometer does not measure time.

5. Freckled is not a hair color.

6. Sled is not construction equipment.

7. Slingshot is not a gun.

8. Tibia is not a finger.

9. Acorns are not a grain.

10. Appointment is not a time period

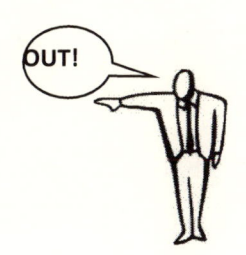

NAME THE ONE THAT DOES NOT BELONG

1. carrot, potato, onion, lettuce

2. tuxedo, blouse, skirt, dress

3. hope, love, sorrow, glee

4. teen, spinster, youth, adolescent

5. hockey, tennis, baseball, football

6. heart, arteries, lungs, veins

7. E, M, O, U

8. library, gym, bedroom, cafeteria

9. grass, sun, beans, peas

10. science, reading, math, gardening

ANSWERS TO: NAME THE ONE THAT DOES NOT BELONG

1. Lettuce is not a root vegetable.

2. Tuxedo is not women's clothing.

3. Sorrow is not a positive feeling.

4. Spinster is not a young person.

5. Hockey is not played with a ball.

6. Lungs are not part of circulation.

7. M is not a vowel.

8. Bedroom is not a room in a school.

9. Sun is not a plant.

10. Gardening is not a school subject.

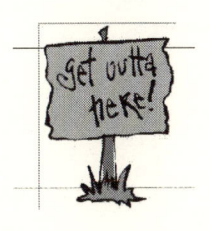

NAME THE ONE THAT DOES NOT BELONG

1. English, Irish, Scotch, Spanish

2. marker, easel, paint, chalk

3. radio, clarinet, drum, flute

4. broccoli, corn, green beans, kale

5. Egypt, Spain, France, Austria

6. seltzer, coke, tonic water, lemonade

7. bird, bee, worm, butterfly

8. knee, elbow, wrist, shin

9. keyboard, mouse, remote, monitor

10. 3, 5, 8, 9

ANSWERS TO: NAME THE ONE THAT DOES NOT BELONG

1. Scotch is not a nationality.

2. Easel is not a drawing tool.

3. Radio is not a musical instrument.

4. Corn is not a green vegetable.

5. Egypt is not a European nation.

6. Lemonade is not a carbonated beverage.

7. Worm cannot fly.

8. Shin cannot bend.

9. Remote is not a computer part.

10. 8 is not an odd number.

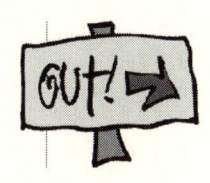

NAME THE ONE THAT DOES **NOT** BELONG

1. helium, marble, oxygen, hydrogen

2. window, telescope, binoculars, oven

3. wail, cry, sob, laugh

4. phone, alarm, microphone, doorbell

5. shout, crawl, walk, run

6. book, magazine, computer, newspaper

7. inspect, view, see, forget

8. cake, ice cream, butter, cheese

9. cashews, pistachios, pecans, popcorn

10. freeze, think, boil, melt

ANSWERS TO: NAME THE ONE THAT DOES <u>NOT</u> BELONG

1. Marble is not an element.

2. Oven is not something we look through.

3. Laugh is not an expression of sadness.

4. Microphone does not ring.

5. Shout does not use legs.

6. Computer is not made of paper.

7. Forget does not involve eyes.

8. Cake is not a dairy product.

9. Popcorn is not a nut.

10. Think is not related to water.

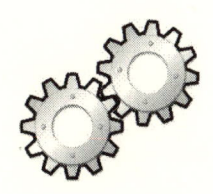

COMPLETE THE COMMON WORD PAIR
(See Appendix for Game Boards A)

1. Church and _____

2. Bear and _____

3. Basketball and _____

4. Syrup and _____

5. Door and _____

6. Diamond and _____

7. Saw and _____

8. Sheets and _____

9. Cheese and _____

10. Dog and _____

11. Needle and _____

12. Helmet and _____

ANSWERS TO: COMPLETE THE COMMON WORD PAIR

1. Church and _____ Steeple _____

2. Bear and _____ Honey _____

3. Basketball and _____ Net, Hoop _____

4. Syrup and _____ Pancakes _____

5. Door and _____ Window _____

6. Diamond and _____ Ring _____

7. Saw and _____ Wood _____

8. Sheets and _____ Bed _____

9. Cheese and _____ Crackers _____

10. Dog and _____ Cat _____

11. Needle and _____ Thread _____

12. Helmet and _____ Motorcycle _____

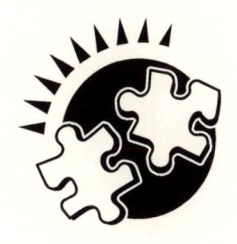

COMPLETE THE COMMON WORD PAIR
(See Appendix for Game Boards B)

1. Bread and _____

2. Coat and _____

3. Comb and _____

4. Cup and _____

5. Salt and _____

6. Nest and _____

7. Ball and _____

8. Macaroni and _____

9. Lock and _____

10. Flashlight and _____

11. Hammer and _____

12. Goldfish and _____

ANSWERS TO: COMPLETE THE COMMON WORD PAIR

1. Bread and   Butter

2. Coat and   Hat

3. Comb and   Hair

4. Cup and   Saucer

5. Salt and   Pepper

6. Nest and   Bird

7. Ball and   Bat

8. Macaroni and   Cheese

9. Lock and   Key

10. Flashlight and   Batteries

11. Hammer and   Nails

12. Goldfish and   Bowl

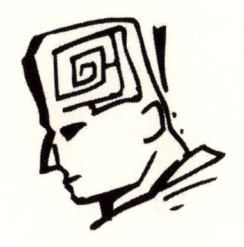

COMPLETE THE COMMON WORD PAIR
(See Appendix for Game Boards C)

1. Chimney and _____

2. Nuts and _____

3. Paint and _____

4. Moon and _____

5. Soap and _____

6. Bank and _____

7. Stars and _____

8. Ladies and _____

9. Acorns and _____

10. Cow and _____

11. Glasses and _____

12. Vase and _____

ANSWERS TO: COMPLETE THE COMMON WORD PAIR

1. Chimney and   Smoke

2. Nuts and   Bolts

3. Paint and   Brush

4. Moon and   Sun

5. Soap and   Water

6. Bank and   Money

7. Stars and   Stripes

8. Ladies and   Gentlemen

9. Acorns and   Squirrel

10. Cow and   Milk

11. Glasses and   Eyes

12. Vase and   Flowers

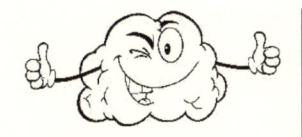

COMPLETE THE COMMON WORD PAIR
(See Appendix for Game Boards D)

1. Meatballs and _____

2. Sheep and _____

3. School and _____

4. Umbrella and _____

5. Ship and _____

6. Lamp and _____

7. Saddle and _____

8. Sleeping Bag and _____

9. Ice Cream and _____

10. Bride and _____

11. Toothpaste and _____

12. Cream and _____

ANSWERS TO: COMPLETE THE COMMON WORD PAIR

1. Meatballs and _____Spaghetti_____

2. Sheep and _____Wool_____

3. School and _____Teacher_____

4. Umbrella and _____Rain_____

5. Ship and _____Sea_____

6. Lamp and _____Shade_____

7. Saddle and _____Horse_____

8. Sleeping Bag and _Tent_____

9. Ice Cream and ___Cone_____

10. Bride and _____Groom_____

11. Toothpaste and _Teeth_____

12. Cream and _____Sugar_____

**COMPLETE THE
COMMON WORD PAIR**
(See Appendix for
Game Boards E)

1. Bee and _____

2. Bib and _____

3. Gifts and _____

4. King and _____

5. Clown and _____

6. Hamburger and _____

7. Fingernail and _____

8. Matches and _____

9. Socks and _____

10. Piano and _____

11. Ink and _____

12. Bow and _____

ANSWERS TO: COMPLETE THE COMMON WORD PAIR

1. Bee and _____ Hive _____

2. Bib and _____ Baby _____

3. Gifts and _____ Birthday _____

4. King and _____ Queen _____

5. Clown and _____ Circus _____

6. Hamburger and _____ Fries _____

7. Fingernail and _____ Polish _____

8. Matches and _____ Fire _____

9. Socks and _____ Shoes _____

10. Piano and _____ Music _____

11. Ink and _____ Pen _____

12. Bow and _____ Arrow _____

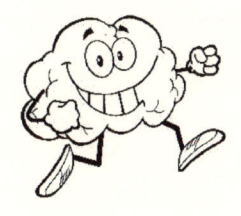

COMPLETE THE COMMON WORD PAIR
(See Appendix for Game Boards F)

1. Pilot and _____

2. Apple and _____

3. Leaves and _____

4. Spider and _____

5. Bacon and _____

6. Peanut Butter and _____

7. Gloves and _____

8. Lion and _____

9. Rocket and _____

10. Witch and _____

11. Duck and _____

12. Baby and _____

ANSWERS TO: COMPLETE THE COMMON WORD PAIR

1. Pilot and _____ Airplane _____

2. Apple and _____ Pie _____

3. Leaves and _____ Tree _____

4. Spider and _____ Web _____

5. Bacon and _____ Eggs _____

6. Peanut Butter and Jelly _____

7. Gloves and _____ Hands _____

8. Lion and _____ Tiger _____

9. Rocket and _____ Moon _____

10. Witch and _____ Broomstick _____

11. Duck and _____ Pond _____

12. Baby and _____ Stroller _____

COMPLETE THE RHYMING WORD PAIR

1. Holy   _____

2. Eensy   _____

3. Itsy   _____

4. Zoot   _____

5. Namby   _____

6. Skinny   _____

7. Thriller   _____

8. Easy   _____

9. Artsy   _____

10. Hootchie   _____

11. Walkie   _____

12. Hob   _____

ANSWERS TO: COMPLETE THE RHYMING WORD PAIR

1. Holy   Moley
2. Eensy   Weensy
3. Itsy   Bitsy
4. Zoot   Suit
5. Namby   Pamby
6. Skinny   Minnie
7. Thriller   Diller
8. Easy   Peasey
9. Artsy   Fartsy
10. Hootchie   Kootchie
11. Walkie   Talkie
12. Hob   Nob

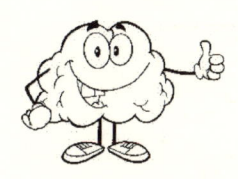

COMPLETE THE RHYMING WORD PAIR

1. Boo   _____

2. Hickory   _____

3. Teeny   _____

4. Willy   _____

5. Fat   _____

6. Handy   _____

7. Fancy   _____

8. Tie   _____

9. Antsy   _____

10. Helter   _____

11. Tootsie   _____

12. Hanky   _____

ANSWERS TO: COMPLETE THE RHYMING WORD PAIR

1. Boo — Hoo
2. Hickory — Dickory
3. Teeny — Weeny
4. Willy — Nilly
5. Fat — Cat
6. Handy — Dandy
7. Fancy — Schmancy
8. Tie — Die
9. Antsy — Pantsy
10. Helter — Skelter
11. Tootsie — Wootsie
12. Hanky — Panky

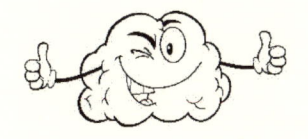

COMPLETE THE RHYMING WORD PAIR

1. Tutti   _____

2. Fuddy   _____

3. Hotsy   _____

4. Local   _____

5. Roley   _____

6. Fuzzy   _____

7. Sneak   _____

8. Motel   _____

9. Itty   _____

10. Footsie   _____

11. Wham   _____

12. Rosy   _____

ANSWERS TO: COMPLETE THE RHYMING WORD PAIR

1. Tutti — Frutti
2. Fuddy — Duddy
3. Hotsy — Totsy
4. Local — Yokel
5. Roley — Poley
6. Fuzzy — Wuzzy
7. Sneak — Peak
8. Motel — No-tell
9. Itty — Bitty
10. Footsie — Wootsie
11. Wham — Bam
12. Rosy — Posey

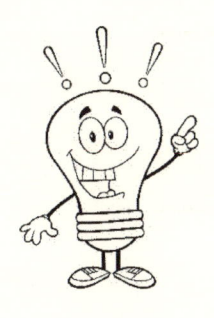

COMPLETE THE RHYMING WORD PAIR

1. Silly _____

2. Okey _____

3. Hum _____

4. Razzle _____

5. Hodge _____

6. Hustle _____

7. Roger _____

8. Poopsie _____

9. Lazy _____

10. Mellow _____

11. Rootin' _____

12. Wheeler _____

ANSWERS TO: COMPLETE THE RHYMING WORD PAIR

1. Silly — Billy
2. Okey — Dokey
3. Hum — Drum
4. Razzle — Dazzle
5. Hodge — Podge
6. Hustle — Bustle
7. Roger — Dodger
8. Poopsie — Woopsie
9. Lazy — Dazy
10. Mellow — Yellow
11. Rootin' — Tootin'
12. Wheeler — Dealer

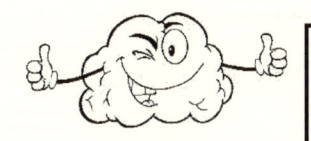

FILL IN THE OPPOSITE WORD

1. Boy and _____

2. War and _____

3. Love and _____

4. Come and _____

5. Heavy and _____

6. Fact and _____

7. Dim and _____

8. Dawn and _____

9. Over and _____

10. Seldom and _____

11. Expensive and _____

12. Succeed and _____

ANSWERS TO: FILL IN THE OPPOSITE WORD

1. Boy and _____Girl_____

2. War and _____Peace_____

3. Love and _____Hate_____

4. Come and _____Go_____

5. Heavy and _____Light_____

6. Fact and _____Fiction_____

7. Dim and _____Bright_____

8. Dawn and _____Dusk_____

9. Over and _____Under_____

10. Seldom and _____Frequently_____

11. Expensive and _____Cheap_____

12. Succeed and _____Fail_____

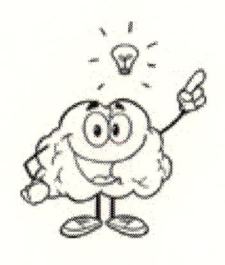

FILL IN THE OPPOSITE WORD

1. Abundant and _____

2. Modern and _____

3. Minimum and _____

4. Pessimist and _____

5. Sow and _____

6. Vain and _____

7. Horizontal and _____

8. Sage and _____

9. Clumsy and _____

10. Opaque and _____

11. Bitter and _____

12. Compulsory and _____

ANSWERS TO: FILL IN THE OPPOSITE WORD

1. Abundant and   Scarce

2. Modern and   Ancient

3. Minimum and   Maximum

4. Pessimist and   Optimist

5. Sow and   Reap

6. Vain and   Humble

7. Horizontal and   Vertical

8. Sage and   Foolish

9. Clumsy and   Graceful

10. Opaque and   Clear

11. Bitter and   Sweet

12. Compulsory and   Voluntary

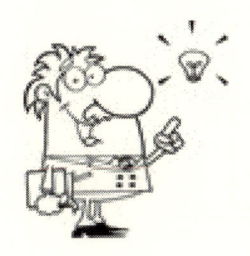

FILL IN THE OPPOSITE WORD

1. Ignorant and _____

2. Worried and _____

3. Grief and _____

4. Interior and _____

5. Identical and _____

6. Artificial and _____

7. Fantasy and _____

8. Hired and _____

9. Teach and _____

10. Offense and _____

11. Servant and _____

12. Refuse and _____

ANSWERS TO: FILL IN THE OPPOSITE WORD

1. Ignorant and   Educated

2. Worried and   Calm

3. Grief and   Joy

4. Interior and   Exterior

5. Identical and   Different

6. Artificial and   Natural

7. Fantasy and   Reality

8. Hired and   Fired

9. Teach and   Learn

10. Offense and   Defense

11. Servant and   Master

12. Refuse and   Accept

FILL IN THE OPPOSITE WORD

1. Boil and _____

2. Silence and _____

3. Question and _____

4. Predator and _____

5. Trap and _____

6. Cease and _____

7. Intentional and _____

8. Admit and _____

9. Comedy and _____

10. Advance and _____

11. Exhibit and _____

12. Forget and _____

ANSWERS TO: FILL IN THE OPPOSITE WORD

1. Boil and _____Freeze_____

2. Silence and _____Noise_____

3. Question and _____Answer_____

4. Predator and _____Prey_____

5. Trap and _____Release_____

6. Cease and _____Begin_____

7. Intentional and _____Accidental_____

8. Admit and _____Deny_____

9. Comedy and _____Tragedy_____

10. Advance and _____Retreat_____

11. Exhibit and _____Conceal_____

12. Forget and _____Remember_____

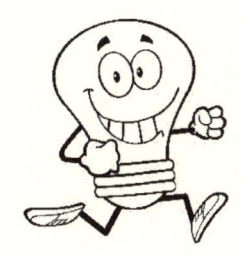

FILL IN THE OPPOSITE WORD

1. Imprison and _____

2. Naked and _____

3. Literal and _____

4. Positive and _____

5. Reward and _____

6. Grin and _____

7. Include and _____

8. Sane and _____

9. Simple and _____

10. Stranger and _____

11. Whisper and _____

12. Strengthen and _____

ANSWERS TO: FILL IN THE OPPOSITE WORD

1. Imprison and _____Free_____

2. Naked and _____Clothed_____

3. Literal and _____Figurative_____

4. Positive and _____Negative_____

5. Reward and _____Punishment_____

6. Grin and _____Frown_____

7. Include and _____Exclude_____

8. Sane and _____Crazy_____

9. Simple and _____Complicated_____

10. Stranger and _____Friend_____

11. Whisper and _____Shout_____

12. Strengthen and _____Weaken_____

FILL IN THE OPPOSITE WORD

1. Doff and _____

2. Shiny and _____

3. Timid and _____

4. Limp and _____

5. Turbulent and _____

6. Imaginary and _____

7. Sparse and _____

8. True and _____

9. Crooked and _____

10. Internal and _____

11. Ceiling and _____

12. Thick and _____

ANSWERS TO: FILL IN THE OPPOSITE WORD

1. Doff and   Don

2. Shiny and   Dull

3. Timid and   Brazen

4. Limp and   Firm

5. Turbulent and   Calm

6. Imaginary and   Real

7. Sparse and   Dense

8. True and   False

9. Crooked and   Straight

10. Internal and   External

11. Ceiling and   Floor

12. Thick and   Thin

FILL IN THE SYNONYM

1. Solution and _____

2. Large and _____

3. Destroy and _____

4. Quick and _____

5. Gift and _____

6. Create and _____

7. Snooze and _____

8. Rip and _____

9. Happy and _____

10. Mad and _____

11. House and _____

12. Chair and _____

ANSWERS TO: FILL IN THE SYNONYM

1. Solution and _____Answer_____

2. Large and _____Big_____

3. Destroy and _____Ruin_____

4. Quick and _____Fast_____

5. Gift and _____Present_____

6. Create and _____Make_____

7. Snooze and _____Sleep_____

8. Rip and _____Tear_____

9. Happy and _____Glad_____

10. Mad and _____Angry_____

11. House and _____Home_____

12. Chair and _____Seat_____

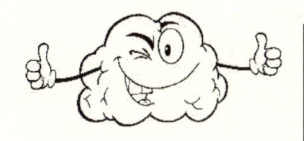

FILL IN THE SYNONYM

1. Awkward and _____

2. Exhausted and _____

3. Attractive and _____

4. Leap and _____

5. Reply and _____

6. Purchase and _____

7. Construct and _____

8. Weep and _____

9. Locate and _____

10. Frighten and _____

11. Odor and _____

12. Beverage and _____

ANSWERS TO: FILL IN THE SYNONYM

1. Awkward and   Clumsy

2. Exhausted and   Tired

3. Attractive and   Handsome

4. Leap and   Jump

5. Reply and   Answer

6. Purchase and   Buy

7. Construct and   Build

8. Weep and   Cry

9. Locate and   Find

10. Frighten and   Scare

11. Odor and   Smell

12. Beverage and   Drink

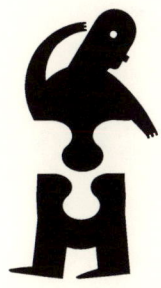

FILL IN THE SYNONYM

1. Abundant and _____

2. Enormous and _____

3. Loyal and _____

4. Perilous and _____

5. Vacant and _____

6. Hilarious and _____

7. Unbiased and _____

8. Fortunate and _____

9. Optimistic and _____

10. Trustworthy and _____

11. Indolent and _____

12. Tyrannical and _____

ANSWERS TO: FILL IN THE SYNONYM

1. Abundant and ___Plentiful___

2. Enormous and ___Gigantic___

3. Loyal and ___Faithful___

4. Perilous and ___Dangerous___

5. Vacant and ___Empty___

6. Hilarious and ___Hysterical___

7. Unbiased and ___Impartial___

8. Fortunate and ___Lucky___

9. Optimistic and ___Positive___

10. Trustworthy and ___Honest___

11. Indolent and ___Lazy___

12. Tyrannical and ___Bossy___

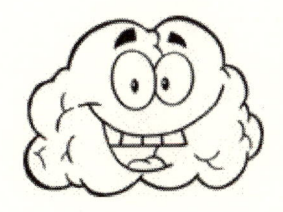

FILL IN THE SYNONYM

1. Merciful and _____

2. Squabble and _____

3. Aperture and _____

4. Adhere and _____

5. Chronic and _____

6. Heal and _____

7. Scowl and _____

8. Lethargic and _____

9. Candid and _____

10. Fragrance and _____

11. Trick and _____

12. Fate and _____

ANSWERS TO: FILL IN THE SYNONYM

1. Merciful and   Compassionate

2. Squabble and   Argue

3. Aperture and   Opening

4. Adhere and   Stick

5. Chronic and   Habitual

6. Heal and   Cure

7. Scowl and   Frown

8. Lethargic and   Sluggish

9. Candid and   Frank

10. Fragrance and   Aroma

11. Trick and   Fool

12. Fate and   Destiny

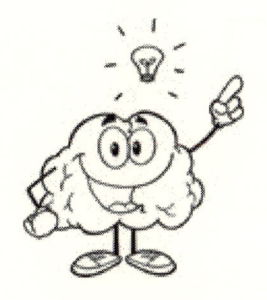

FILL IN THE SYNONYM

1. Obese and _____

2. Fatigue and _____

3. Equipment and _____

4. Conquer and _____

5. Scorch and _____

6. Obstruct and _____

7. Suggest and _____

8. Persist and _____

9. Repose and _____

10. Display and _____

11. Topic and _____

12. Authentic and _____

ANSWERS TO: FILL IN THE SYNONYM

1. Obese and _____Fat_____

2. Fatigue and _____Tire_____

3. Equipment and _____Gear_____

4. Conquer and _____Defeat_____

5. Scorch and _____Burn_____

6. Obstruct and _____Hinder_____

7. Suggest and _____Hint_____

8. Persist and _____Persevere_____

9. Repose and _____Rest_____

10. Display and _____Show_____

11. Topic and _____Subject_____

12. Authentic and _____Genuine_____

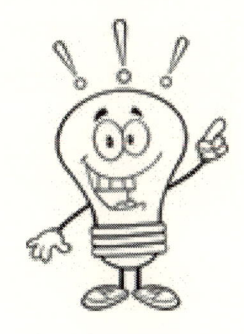

FILL IN THE SYNONYM

1. Audacious and _____

2. Promise and _____

3. Forecast and _____

4. Placate and _____

5. Tidy and _____

6. Ethical and _____

7. Resemblance and _____

8. Immaterial and _____

9. Imitate and _____

10. Pliable and _____

11. Oust and _____

12. Extol and _____

ANSWERS TO: FILL IN THE SYNONYM

1. Audacious and   Bold

2. Promise and   Vow

3. Forecast and   Predict

4. Placate and   Pacify

5. Tidy and   Neat

6. Ethical and   Moral

7. Resemblance and   Similarity

8. Immaterial and   Irrelevant

9. Imitate and   Copy

10. Pliable and   Flexible

11. Oust and   Expel

12. Extol and   Praise

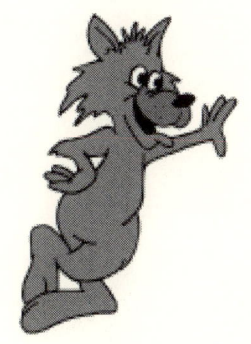

FILL IN THE CARTOON CHARACTER

1. Popeye and _____

2. Mickey Mouse and _____

3. Peter Pan and _____

4. Batman and _____

5. Donald Duck and _____

6. Pinocchio and _____

7. Lady and _____

8. Mutt and _____

9. Chip and _____

10. Beavis and _____

11. Snoopy and _____

12. Rocky and _____

ANSWERS TO: FILL IN THE CARTOON CHARACTER

1. Popeye and _____Olive Oyl_____

2. Mickey Mouse and _Minnie_____

3. Peter Pan and _____Wendy_____

4. Batman and _____Robin_____

5. Donald Duck and _Daisy_____

6. Pinocchio and _____Jiminy Cricket_____

7. Lady and _____The Tramp_____

8. Mutt and _____Jeff_____

9. Chip and _____Dale_____

10. Beavis and _____Butthead_____

11. Snoopy and _____Charlie Brown_____

12. Rocky and _____Bullwinkle_____

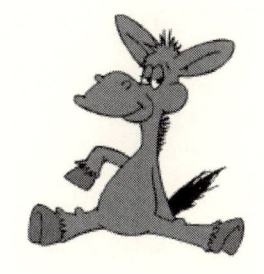

FILL IN THE CARTOON CHARACTER

1. Pooh and _____

2. Sylvester and _____

3. Lois Lane and _____

4. Miss Piggy and _____

5. Fred Flintstone and _____

6. Bert and _____

7. Tom and _____

8. Archie and _____

9. Snow White and _____

10. Puss and _____

11. Tweedledum and _____

12. Raggedy Ann and _____

ANSWERS TO: FILL IN THE CARTOON CHARACTER

1. Pooh and __Tigger__

2. Sylvester and __Tweety__

3. Lois Lane and __Superman__

4. Miss Piggy and __Kermit__

5. Fred Flintstone and __Wilma__

6. Bert and __Ernie__

7. Tom and __Jerry__

8. Archie and __Jughead__

9. Snow White and __Seven Dwarves__

10. Puss and __Boots__

11. Tweedledum and __Tweedledee__

12. Raggedy Ann and __Andy__

COMPLETE THE FAMOUS DUO

1. Anthony and _____

2. Mork and _____

3. Ozzie and _____

4. Amos and _____

5. Abbot and _____

6. Fred Astaire and _____

7. Roy Rogers and _____

8. Romeo and _____

9. Adam and _____

10. Sonny and _____

11. Jekyll and _____

12. David and _____

ANSWERS TO: COMPLETE THE FAMOUS DUO

1. Anthony and _____Cleopatra_____

2. Mork and _____Mindy_____

3. Ozzie and _____Harriet_____

4. Amos and _____Andy_____

5. Abbot and _____Costello_____

6. Fred Astaire and _____Ginger Rogers_____

7. Roy Rogers and _____Dale Evans_____

8. Romeo and _____Juliet_____

9. Adam and _____Eve_____

10. Sonny and _____Sher_____

11. Jekyll and _____Hyde_____

12. David and _____Goliath_____

COMPLETE THE FAMOUS DUO

1. Laverne and _____

2. Desi and _____

3. Laurel and _____

4. Lone Ranger and _____

5. Starsky and _____

6. Cheech and _____

7. Tarzan and _____

8. Cain and _____

9. Samson and _____

10. Robin Hood and _____

11. Barbie and _____

12. John Smith and _____

ANSWERS TO: COMPLETE THE FAMOUS DUO

1. Laverne and _Shirley_

2. Desi and _Lucy_

3. Laurel and _Hardy_

4. Lone Ranger and _Tonto_

5. Starsky and _Hutch_

6. Cheech and _Chong_

7. Tarzan and _Jane_

8. Cain and _Abel_

9. Samson and _Delilah_

10. Robin Hood and _Maid Marion_

11. Barbie and _Ken_

12. John Smith and _Pocahontas_

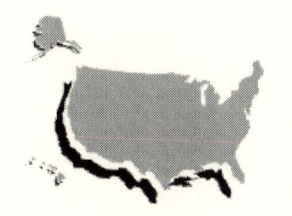

COMPLETE THE STATE CAPITAL

1. Sacramento, _____

2. Boston, _____

3. Austin, _____

4. Montgomery, _____

5. Juneau, _____

6. Atlanta, _____

7. Jefferson City, _____

8. Helena, _____

9. Annapolis, _____

10. St. Paul, _____

11. Augusta, _____

12. Jackson, _____

ANSWERS TO: COMPLETE THE STATE CAPITAL

1. Sacramento, _____California_____

2. Boston, _____Massachusetts_____

3. Austin, _____Texas_____

4. Montgomery, _____Alabama_____

5. Juneau, _____Alaska_____

6. Atlanta, _____Georgia_____

7. Jefferson City, _____Missouri_____

8. Helena, _____Montana_____

9. Annapolis, _____Maryland_____

10. St. Paul, _____Minnesota_____

11. Augusta, _____Maine_____

12. Jackson, _____Mississippi_____

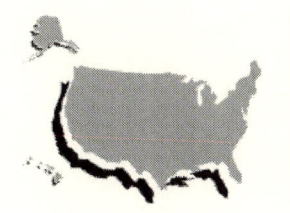

COMPLETE THE STATE CAPITAL

1. Little Rock, _____

2. Denver, _____

3. Hartford, _____

4. Lansing, _____

5. Dover, _____

6. Concord, _____

7. Tallahassee, _____

8. Boise, _____

9. Baton Rouge, _____

10. Charleston, _____

11. Trenton, _____

12. Topeka, _____

ANSWERS TO: COMPLETE THE STATE CAPITAL

1. Little Rock, _____Arkansas_____

2. Denver, _____Colorado_____

3. Hartford, _____Connecticut_____

4. Lansing, _____Michigan_____

5. Dover, _____Delaware_____

6. Concord, _____New Hampshire_____

7. Tallahassee, _____Florida_____

8. Boise, _____Idaho_____

9. Baton Rouge, _____Louisiana_____

10. Charleston, _____West Virginia_____

11. Trenton, _____New Jersey_____

12. Topeka, _____Kansas_____

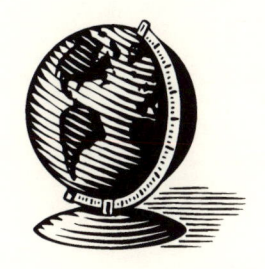

COMPLETE THE NATIONAL CAPITAL

1. Santiago, _____

2. Cairo, _____

3. Kabul, _____

4. New Delhi, _____

5. Copenhagen, _____

6. Lisbon, _____

7. Ottawa, _____

8. Kingston, _____

9. London, _____

10. Nairobi, _____

11. Phnom Penh, _____

12. Bern, _____

ANSWERS TO: COMPLETE THE NATIONAL CAPITAL

1. Santiago, Chile

2. Cairo, Egypt

3. Kabul, Afghanistan

4. New Delhi, India

5. Copenhagen, Denmark

6. Lisbon, Portugal

7. Ottawa, Canada

8. Kingston, Jamaica

9. London, England

10. Nairobi, Kenya

11. Phnom Penh, Cambodia

12. Bern, Switzerland

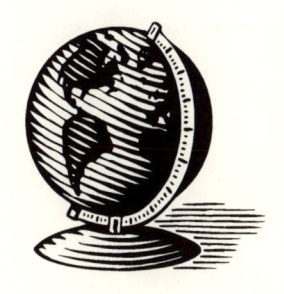

COMPLETE THE NATIONAL CAPITAL

1. Addis Ababa, _____

2. Beijing, _____

3. Baghdad, _____

4. Vienna, _____

5. Warsaw, _____

6. Nassau, _____

7. Santo Domingo, _____

8. Port-au-Prince, _____

9. Buenos Aires, _____

10. Berlin, _____

11. Pretoria, _____

12. Kiev, _____

ANSWERS TO: COMPLETE THE NATIONAL CAPITAL

1. Addis Ababa, Ethiopia

2. Beijing, China

3. Baghdad, Iraq

4. Vienna, Austria

5. Warsaw, Poland

6. Nassau, Bahamas

7. Santo Domingo, Dominican Republic

8. Port-au-Prince, Haiti

9. Buenos Aires, Argentina

10. Berlin, Germany

11. Pretoria, South Africa

12. Kiev, Ukraine

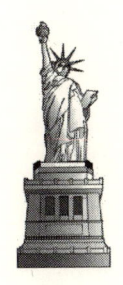

WHERE IS THE FAMOUS PLACE?

1. Badlands, _____

2. Disneyworld, _____

3. Hollywood, _____

4. Yellowstone, _____

5. Grand Canyon, _____

6. The Alamo, _____

7. Niagara Falls, _____

8. Everglades, _____

9. Statue of Liberty, _____

10. Hoover Dam, _____

11. Kennedy Space Center, _____

12. Grand Ole Opry, _____

ANSWERS TO: WHERE IS THE FAMOUS PLACE?

1. Badlands, South Dakota

2. Disneyworld, Florida

3. Hollywood, California

4. Yellowstone, Wyoming

5. Grand Canyon, Arizona

6. The Alamo, Texas

7. Niagara Falls, New York

8. Everglades, Florida

9. Statue of Liberty, New York City

10. Hoover Dam, AZ and NV

11. Kennedy Space Center, Florida

12. Grand Ole Opry, Tennessee

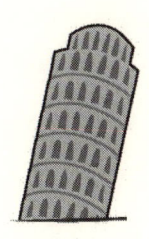

WHERE IS THE FAMOUS PLACE?

1. Eifel Tower, _____

2. Mount Everest, _____

3. Great Pyramid, _____

4. The Great Wall, _____

5. Stonehenge, _____

6. The Leaning Tower, _____

7. Auschwitz, _____

8. Jungfrau, _____

9. Taj Mahal, _____

10. Machu Picchu, _____

11. Great Barrier Reef, _____

12. Chichen Itza, _____

ANSWERS TO: WHERE IS THE FAMOUS PLACE?

1. Eifel Tower, <u>   Paris   </u>

2. Mount Everest, <u> Nepal </u>

3. Great Pyramid, <u> Egypt </u>

4. The Great Wall, <u> China </u>

5. Stonehenge, <u> England </u>

6. The Leaning Tower, <u>Italy</u>

7. Auschwitz, <u> Poland </u>

8. Jungfrau, <u> Switzerland </u>

9. Taj Mahal, <u> India </u>

10. Machu Picchu, <u> Peru </u>

11. Great Barrier Reef, <u>Australia</u>

12. Chichen Itza, <u> Mexico </u>

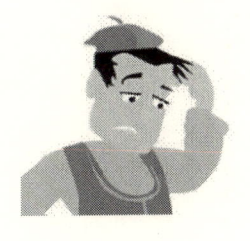

NAME AT LEAST 10 ITEMS IN THE CATEGORY… as fast as you can!

PETS: _____

_____

_____

CLOTHES: _____

_____

_____

FRUITS: _____

_____

_____

VEGETABLES: _____

_____

_____

ANSWERS TO: NAME AT LEAST 10 ITEMS IN THE CATEGORY

PETS: dog, cat, horse, rabbit, turtle, gerbil, pig, guinea pig, parakeet, goldfish, hamster

CLOTHES: hat, coat, dress, shirt, jacket, pants, underwear, skirt, socks, shoes, pajamas, gloves, scarf

FRUITS: apple, pear, peach, grapes, kiwi, watermelon, pineapple, lime, lemon, grapefruit, strawberry

VEGETABLES: peas, beans, corn, potatoes, lettuce, cabbage, spinach, broccoli, brussel sprouts, carrots

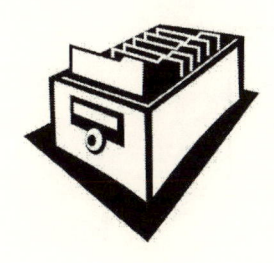

NAME AT LEAST 10 ITEMS IN THE CATEGORY ... as fast as you can!

SPORTS: _____

_____

_____

APPLIANCES: _____

_____

_____

FURNITURE: _____

_____

_____

COLORS: _____

_____

_____

ANSWERS TO: NAME AT LEAST 10 ITEMS IN THE CATEGORY

SPORTS: hockey, baseball, golf, tennis, swimming, football, soccer, basketball, skiing, volleyball

APPLIANCES: blender, can opener, fridge, dishwasher, stove, waffle iron, mixer, toaster, microwave, coffee pot

FURNITURE: desk, sofa, dresser, table, chair, ottoman, bookcase, coffee table, credenza, cabinet

COLORS: red, blue, yellow, purple, black, brown, orange, tan, white, violet

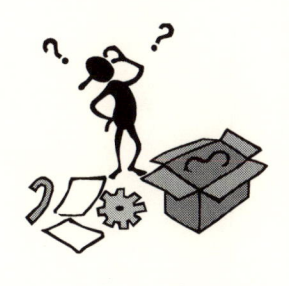

NAME AT LEAST 10 ITEMS IN THE CATEGORY... as fast as you can!

BEVERAGES: _____

_____

_____

DESSERTS: _____

_____

_____

PRESIDENTS: _____

_____

_____

ZOO ANIMALS: _____

_____

_____

ANSWERS TO: NAME AT LEAST 10 ITEMS IN THE CATEGORY

BEVERAGES: milk, soda, coffee, tea, lemonade, juice, water, seltzer, wine, beer

DESSERTS: pie, cake, custard, pudding, ice cream, parfait, brownie, cheesecake, cobbler, tart

PRESIDENTS: Washington, Grant, Lincoln, Nixon, Kennedy, Johnson, Bush, Adams, Ford, Reagan, Clinton

ZOO ANIMALS: lion, tiger, zebra, monkey, gorilla, hippo, rhino, giraffe, elephant, penguin

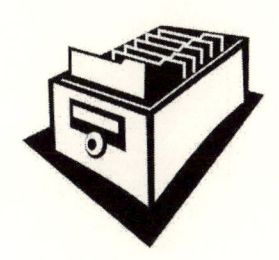

NAME AT LEAST 10 ITEMS IN THE CATEGORY... as fast as you can!

VEHICLES: _____

_____

_____

FARM ANIMALS: _____

_____

_____

MUSICAL INSTRUMENTS: _____

_____

_____

FISH: _____

_____

_____

ANSWERS TO: NAME AT LEAST 10 ITEMS IN THE CATEGORY

VEHICLES: car, truck, tractor, train, plane, helicopter, van, subway, ambulance, fire engine

FARM ANIMALS: goat, cow, sheep, pig, horse, chicken, rooster, duck, ox, donkey

MUSICAL INSTRUMENTS: piano, guitar, violin, harmonica, accordion, drum, saxophone, clarinet, flute, oboe

FISH: shark, tuna, carp, perch, cod, trout, salmon, mackerel, bluefish, bass, minnow

GROUP A

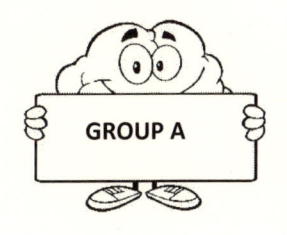

NAME AT LEAST 10 ITEMS IN THE CATEGORY... as fast as you can!

OCCUPATIONS: _____

_____

_____

CARPENTER'S TOOLS: _____

_____

_____

BIRDS: _____

_____

_____

INSECTS: _____

_____

_____

ANSWERS TO: NAME AT LEAST 10 ITEMS IN THE CATEGORY

OCCUPATIONS: doctor, lawyer, nurse, carpenter, electrician, plumber, secretary, teacher, engineer, chef

CARPENTER'S TOOLS: hammer, tape measure, screwdriver, drill, saw, level, chisel, pliers, putty knife, wrench

BIRDS: hawk, eagle, blue jay, bluebird, robin, sparrow, wren, crow, blackbird, falcon

INSECTS: ladybug, beetle, cricket, ant, grub, flea, grasshopper, bumblebee, moth, dragonfly

???

NAME THE CATEGORY

1. lemonade, milk, water, seltzer

2. lawyer, nurse, plumber, custodian

3. diamond, ruby, emerald, sapphire

4. ring, watch, bracelet, necklace

5. car, truck, taxi, ambulance

6. petals, stems, roots, leaves

7. cob, husk, kernels, stalk

8. sour, sweet, bitter, salty

9. wheel, windshield, muffler, engine

10. scissors, ax, knife, saw

ANSWERS TO: NAME THE CATEGORY

1. beverages, drinks

2. occupations, jobs

3. jewels, gems

4. jewelry

5. vehicles

6. parts of a flower

7. parts of corn

8. flavors, tastes

9. parts of a car

10. tools that cut

???

NAME THE CATEGORY

1. uncle, cousin, grandfather, sister

2. circulatory, respiratory, digestive, skeletal

3. cube, sphere, cylinder, cone

4. Pacific, Atlantic, Indian, Arctic

5. Europe, Africa, North America, Asia

6. nickel, penny, dime, quarter

7. crab, lobster, oyster, clam

8. hemlock, spruce, cedar, pine

9. ounces, pounds, tons, grams

10. happy, sad, angry, confused

ANSWERS TO: NAME THE CATEGORY

1. relatives

2. systems of the body

3. geometric shapes

4. oceans

5. continents

6. coins

7. shellfish

8. evergreen trees

9. measures of weight

10. feelings

???

NAME THE CATEGORY

1. Venus, Mars, Earth, Jupiter

2. pie, cake, ice cream, pudding

3. slippers, socks, shoes, boots

4. aspirin, antihistamine, laxative, antacid

5. thermometer, barometer, ruler, scale

6. summer, winter, spring, fall

7. Kennedy, Lincoln, Adams, Reagan

8. baseball, soccer, football, tennis

9. igneous, metamorphic, sedimentary

10. Columbus, Magellan, Eriksson, Armstrong

ANSWERS TO: NAME THE CATEGORY

1. planets
2. desserts
3. footwear
4. medicines
5. tools that measure
6. seasons
7. presidents
8. sports
9. rocks
10. explorers

???

NAME THE CATEGORY

1. Thanksgiving, Memorial Day, Labor Day, New Year's Day

2. stove, refrigerator, microwave, dishwasher

3. grater, peeler, spatula, flipper

4. sit-up, pull-up, push-up, jumping jack

5. fragrant, musky, pungent, stinky

6. cerebrum, cerebellum, cortex, frontal lobe

7. measles, mumps, chicken pox, polio

8. capellini, fusilli, ziti, spaghetti

9. clarinet, saxophone, trumpet, trombone

10. fingers, toes, worms, jello

ANSWERS TO: NAME THE CATEGORY

1. holidays

2. appliances

3. utensils

4. exercises

5. scents

6. parts of the brain

7. diseases

8. pasta

9. horns, wind instruments

10. things that wiggle

???

NAME THE CATEGORY

1. deltoid, trapezius, biceps, triceps

2. Bach, Chopin, Brahms, Beethoven

3. math, science, art, history

4. cotton, linen, silk, rayon

5. mayonnaise, mustard, wasabi, ketchup

6. cinnamon, sage, thyme, basil

7. M, K, Q, R

8. Cancer, Libra, Virgo, Taurus

9. Orion, Pegasus, Ursa Major, Ursa Minor

10. north, south, southwest, east

ANSWERS TO: NAME THE CATEGORY

1. muscles

2. composers

3. school subjects

4. fabric

5. condiments

6. spices

7. consonant letters

8. astrological signs

9. constellations

10. directions

???

NAME THE CATEGORY

1. Monday, Friday, Saturday, Tuesday

2. Jane, Bridget, Mary, Susan

3. girl, lady, mother, woman

4. blocks, puzzles, dolls, marbles

5. Ohio, Florida, Utah, Michigan

6. inches, yards, miles, feet

7. X, L, V, C

8. Wow! Oh no! Yikes! Hooray!

9. Nile, Amazon, Thames, Mississippi

10. wheat, rye, oats, barley

ANSWERS TO: NAME THE CATEGORY

1. days of the week

2. girls' names

3. female terms

4. toys

5. states

6. measures of length or distance

7. Roman numerals

8. exclamations

9. rivers

10. grains

???

NAME THE CATEGORY

1. March, June, July, September

2. Bob, Chip, Jack, George

3. arm, leg, head, finger

4. cow, duck, chicken, pig

5. chords, lyrics, notes, rhythm

6. neapolitan, vanilla, strawberry, pistachio

7. rain, snow, hail, sleet

8. Judaism, Christianity, Islam, Buddhism

9. blonde, brunette, auburn, gray

10. pound, peso, euro, dinar

ANSWERS TO: NAME THE CATEGORY

1. months

2. boys' names

3. body parts

4. farm animals

5. musical terms

6. ice cream flavors

7. precipitation

8. religions

9. hair colors

10. currencies, money

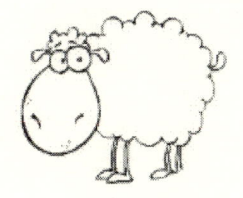

NAME THE ANIMAL'S YOUNG

1. Cow and _____

2. Bear and _____

3. Frog and _____

4. Cat and _____

5. Dog and _____

6. Bird and _____

7. Owl and _____

8. Butterfly and _____

9. Deer and _____

10. Giraffe and _____

11. Duck and _____

12. Elephant and _____

ANSWERS TO: NAME THE ANIMAL'S YOUNG

1. Cow and _____ Calf _____

2. Bear and _____ Cub _____

3. Frog and _____ Tadpole _____

4. Cat and _____ Kitten _____

5. Dog and _____ Puppy _____

6. Bird and _____ Chick _____

7. Owl and _____ Owlet _____

8. Butterfly and _____ Caterpillar _____

9. Deer and _____ Fawn _____

10. Giraffe and _____ Calf _____

11. Duck and _____ Duckling _____

12. Elephant and _____ Calf _____

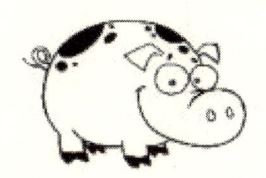

NAME THE ANIMAL'S YOUNG

1. Fly and _____

2. Goat and _____

3. Goose and _____

4. Horse and _____

5. Kangaroo and _____

6. Lion and _____

7. Fish and _____

8. Pig and _____

9. Sheep and _____

10. Swan and _____

11. Rabbit and _____

12. Whale and _____

ANSWERS TO: NAME THE ANIMAL'S YOUNG

1. Fly and _____Maggot_____

2. Goat and _____Kid_____

3. Goose and _____Gosling_____

4. Horse and __Pony, Foal, Colt, Filly__

5. Kangaroo and _____Joey_____

6. Lion and _____Cub_____

7. Fish and _____Fry_____

8. Pig and _____Piglet_____

9. Sheep and _____Lamb_____

10. Swan and _____Cygnet_____

11. Rabbit and _____Kit_____

12. Whale and _____Calf_____

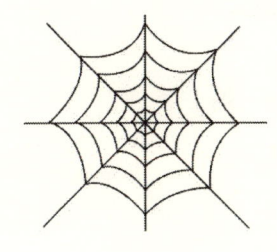

NAME THE ANIMAL'S HOME

1. Bee and _____

2. Rabbit and _____

3. Dog and _____

4. Whale and _____

5. Chicken and _____

6. Pig and _____

7. Cow and _____

8. Horse and _____

9. Spider and _____

10. Ant and _____

11. Bird and _____

12. Snake and _____

ANSWERS TO: NAME THE ANIMAL'S HOME

1. Bee and _____ Hive _____

2. Rabbit and _____ Hutch, Burrow _____

3. Dog and _____ Kennel, House _____

4. Whale and _____ Sea, Ocean _____

5. Chicken and _____ Coop _____

6. Pig and _____ Pen, Sty _____

7. Cow and _____ Barn, Shed _____

8. Horse and _____ Stable, Stall _____

9. Spider and _____ Web _____

10. Ant and _____ Hill, Farm, Nest _____

11. Bird and _____ Cage, Nest _____

12. Snake and _____ Hole _____

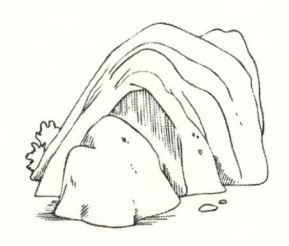

NAME THE ANIMAL'S HOME

1. Turtle and _____

2. Monkey and _____

3. Penguin and _____

4. Squirrel and _____

5. Termite and _____

6. Panda and _____

7. Bat and _____

8. Bear and _____

9. Camel and _____

10. Lion and _____

11. Mouse and _____

12. Duck and _____

ANSWERS TO: NAME THE ANIMAL'S HOME

1. Turtle and   Sea

2. Monkey and   Tree

3. Penguin and   Rookery

4. Squirrel and   Drey, Nest

5. Termite and   Mound

6. Panda and   Bamboo Tree

7. Bat and   Cave, Roost

8. Bear and   Cave

9. Camel and   Desert

10. Lion and   Den, Lair

11. Mouse and   Hole

12. Duck and   Pond

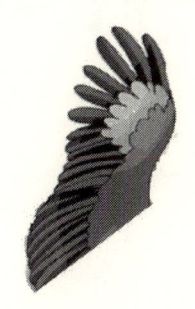

WHAT ANIMAL HAS THIS PART?

1. _____snout_____

2. _____stinger_____

3. _____utters_____

4. _____horns_____

5. _____mane_____

6. _____pouch_____

7. _____gills_____

8. _____shell_____

9. _____blowhole_____

10. _____antlers_____

ANSWERS TO: WHAT ANIMAL HAS THIS PART?

1. pig
2. bee, wasp
3. cow
4. bull, ox
5. horse, lion
6. kangaroo
7. fish
8. turtle, fish
9. whale
10. deer, moose

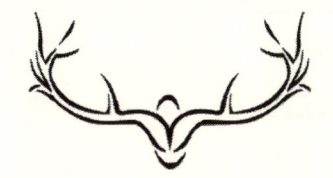

WHAT ANIMAL HAS THIS PART?

1. _____ tusk _____

2. _____ talon _____

3. _____ comb _____

4. _____ trunk _____

5. _____ bill _____

6. _____ hump _____

7. _____ hoof _____

8. _____ beak _____

9. _____ quill _____

10. _____ wool _____

ANSWERS TO: WHAT ANIMAL HAS THIS PART?

1. rhino, elephant

2. eagle, hawk

3. rooster

4. elephant

5. duck

6. camel

7. horse, cow

8. bird

9. porcupine

10. sheep

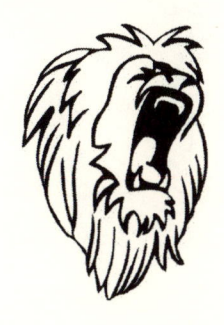

WHAT ANIMAL MAKES THIS SOUND?

1. _____ moo _____

2. _____ gobble _____

3. _____ bark _____

4. _____ bleat _____

5. _____ whinny _____

6. _____ cluck _____

7. _____ coo _____

8. _____ roar _____

9. _____ bray _____

10. _____ mew _____

ANSWERS TO: WHAT ANIMAL MAKES THIS SOUND?

1. cow
2. turkey
3. dog
4. sheep, goat
5. horse
6. chicken
7. dove
8. lion
9. donkey
10. cat

WHAT ANIMAL MAKES THIS SOUND?

1. _____ squeal _____

2. _____ hiss _____

3. _____ quack _____

4. _____ chirp _____

5. _____ hoot _____

6. _____ caw _____

7. _____ peep _____

8. _____ howl _____

9. _____ honk _____

10. _____ croak _____

ANSWERS TO: WHAT ANIMAL MAKES THIS SOUND?

1. pig
2. snake
3. duck
4. bird, cricket
5. owl
6. crow
7. chick
8. wolf, coyote
9. goose
10. frog

NAME SOMETHING ....

1. that rips _____

2. that stings _____

3. that cuts _____

4. that rises _____

5. that shatters _____

6. that whistles _____

7. that fastens _____

8. that ties _____

9. that flashes _____

10. that rings _____

ANSWERS TO: NAME SOMETHING ....

1. paper, fabric, cardboard, foil, cloth

2. bee, jellyfish, needle, ant, burn

3. scissors, knife, saw, razor, ax, mower

4. sun, balloon, dough, moon, stock market

5. glass, window, windshield

6. train, whistle, teapot

7. button, zipper, Velcro, string, rope, tape, glue

8. ribbon, string, rope, shoelaces, necktie, scarf

9. light, lightning, alarm

10. bell, timer, alarm, elevator, phone, doorbell

NAME SOMETHING ....

1. that roars   _____

2. that shines   _____

3. that drips   _____

4. that colors   _____

5. that writes   _____

6. that pinches   _____

7. that cooks   _____

8. that flies   _____

9. that measures   _____

10. that ticks   _____

ANSWERS TO: NAME SOMETHING ....

1. lion, tiger, fire, furnace, volcano
2. sun, moon, star, diamond, light, silver
3. nose, faucet, hose, pipe
4. crayon, marker, paint, dye, pencil
5. pen, pencil, typewriter, computer printer
6. fingers, bug, crab, tweezers, tongs, lobster
7. fire, oven, stove, grill, microwave
8. bird, plane, kite, balloon, butterfly, bug
9. ruler, scale, thermometer, barometer, yardstick
10. clock, bomb, timer, heart

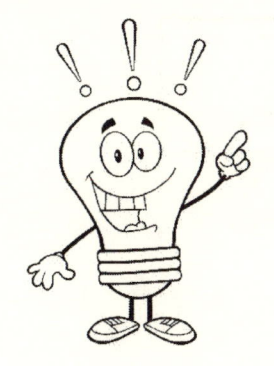

NAME SOMETHING ....

1. that crawls _____

2. that melts _____

3. that squeaks _____

4. that pops _____

5. that grows _____

6. that burns _____

7. that cleans _____

8. that lays eggs_____

9. that rotates _____

10. that deflates _____

ANSWERS TO: NAME SOMETHING ....

1. baby, turtle, ant, bug

2. ice, ice cream, glacier, chocolate

3. mouse, springs, stairs, floor, brakes

4. bubble, balloon, popcorn, jack-in-the-box

5. person, plant, animal, wealth, garden

6. fire, match, stove, sun, candle, flame

7. vacuum, broom, mop, rag, sponge, brush

8. chicken, bird, turtle, snake, alligator, crocodile

9. wheel, propeller, gear, globe, windmill, top

10. balloon, tire, ego, tube, float, raft

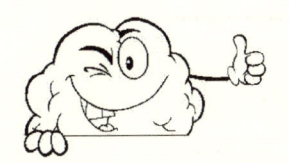

NAME SOMETHING ....

1. you pour _____

2. you open _____

3. you read _____

4. you watch _____

5. you twist _____

6. you light _____

7. you cut _____

8. you chew _____

9. you bake _____

10. you insure _____

ANSWERS TO: NAME SOMETHING ....

1. milk, soda, water, coffee

2. door, window, book, letter, present, cupboard

3. book, newspaper, magazine, email, mail

4. TV, parade, sporting event, play, opera, performance

5. lid, doorknob, ankle, lightbulb, pepper mill

6. fire, match, candle, grill

7. paper, cloth, fabric, wood, logs, trees, flowers

8. food, gum, tobacco

9. cake, cookies, pie, casserole, fish, chicken

10. car, home, jewelry, health, boat, mortgage

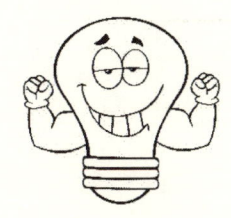

NAME A WORD THAT DESCRIBES ...

1. feather

2. ox

3. rose

4. diamond

5. comedian

6. clown

7. motorcycle

8. cloud

9. cactus

10. ice

11. fox

12. wheel

ANSWERS TO: NAME A WORD THAT DESCRIBES ...

1. feather — light, soft
2. ox — strong, dumb
3. rose — sweet, fragrant
4. diamond — sparkly, expensive
5. comedian — funny
6. clown — silly
7. motorcycle — fast, dangerous, noisy
8. cloud — puffy, white, dark
9. cactus — prickly
10. ice — frozen, cold
11. fox — sly
12. wheel — round

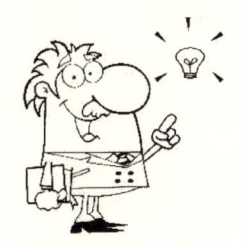

NAME A WORD THAT DESCRIBES …

1. jello

2. gum

3. sun

4. summer

5. winter

6. millionaire

7. pauper

8. lion

9. mouse

10. zebra

11. fire

12. baby

ANSWERS TO: NAME A WORD THAT DESCRIBES ...

1. jello — wiggly
2. gum — sticky, chewy
3. sun — hot, bright
4. summer — hot
5. winter — cold
6. millionaire — rich
7. pauper — poor
8. lion — mighty, fierce
9. mouse — timid, quiet
10. zebra — striped
11. fire — hot, smoky
12. baby — cute

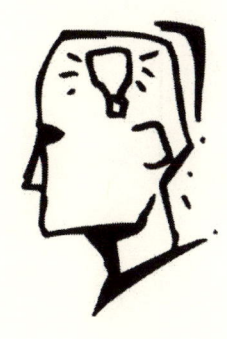

NAME A WORD THAT DESCRIBES ...

1. knife
2. dog
3. mountain
4. ball
5. snow
6. rain
7. Marilyn Monroe
8. lemon
9. boulder
10. cotton candy
11. roller coaster
12. thunder

ANSWERS TO: NAME A WORD THAT DESCRIBES …

1. knife — sharp
2. dog — loyal, soft
3. mountain — steep
4. ball — round, bouncy
5. snow — cold, white
6. rain — wet
7. Marilyn Monroe — blonde, sexy
8. lemon — sour
9. boulder — heavy, hard
10. cotton candy — sweet, sticky
11. roller coaster — fast, scary
12. thunder — loud

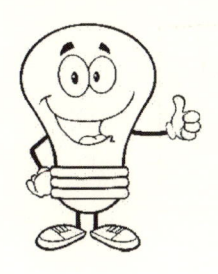

NAME A WORD THAT DESCRIBES ...

1. witch
2. friend
3. professor
4. worm
5. garbage
6. monster
7. ballerina
8. cave
9. river
10. silk
11. pig
12. crystal

ANSWERS TO: NAME A WORD THAT DESCRIBES ...

1. witch — ugly, scary
2. friend — loyal, fun, good
3. professor — smart, absent-minded
4. worm — wiggly, squishy
5. garbage — stinky, yucky
6. monster — scary
7. ballerina — graceful, pretty
8. cave — dark, damp
9. river — winding, wide, deep
10. silk — smooth
11. pig — fat, dirty, muddy
12. crystal — clear

FIND 6 COMPOUND WORDS
(words comprised of 2 smaller words; e.g. "ear" and "ring" is "earring")

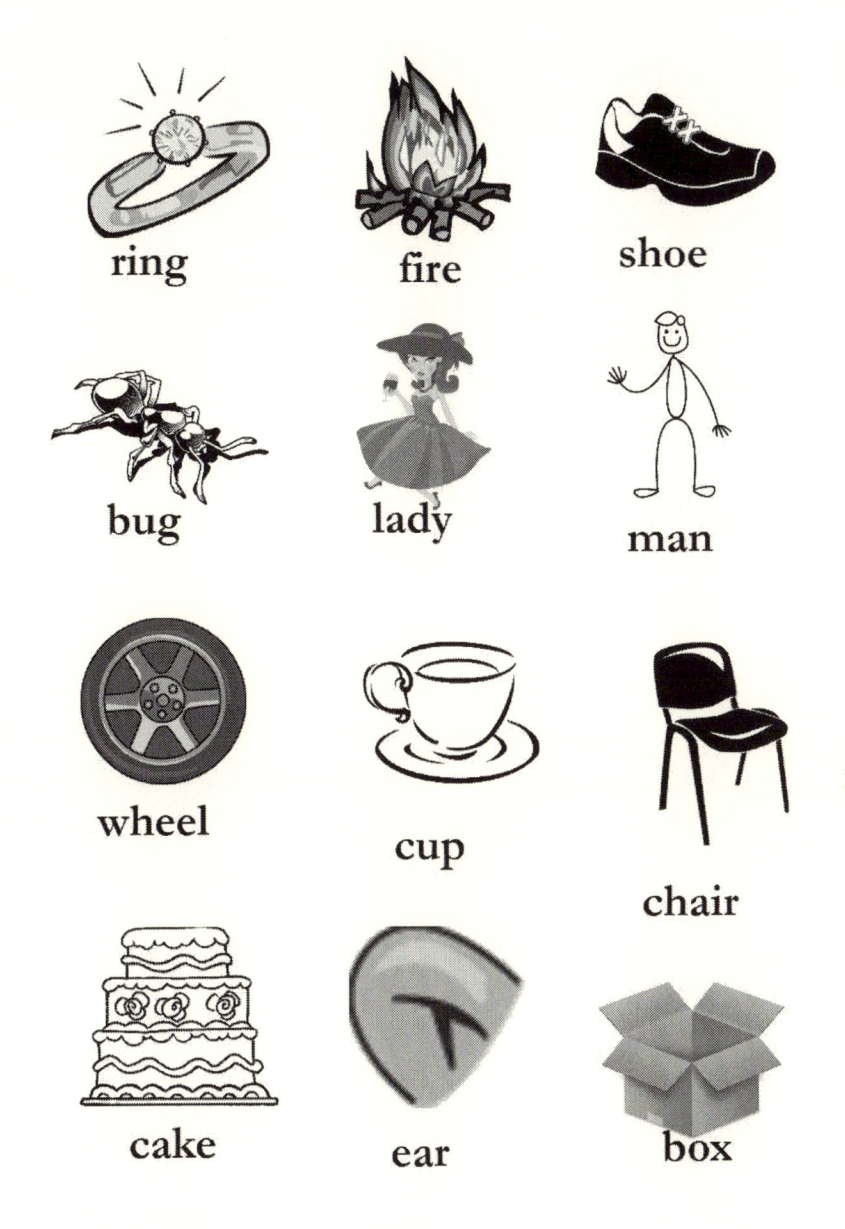

ring	fire	shoe
bug	lady	man
wheel	cup	chair
cake	ear	box

ANSWERS TO: FIND 6 COMPOUND WORDS

1. _____earring_____

2. _____fireman_____

3. _____shoebox_____

4. _____ladybug_____

5. _____wheelchair_____

6. _____cupcake_____

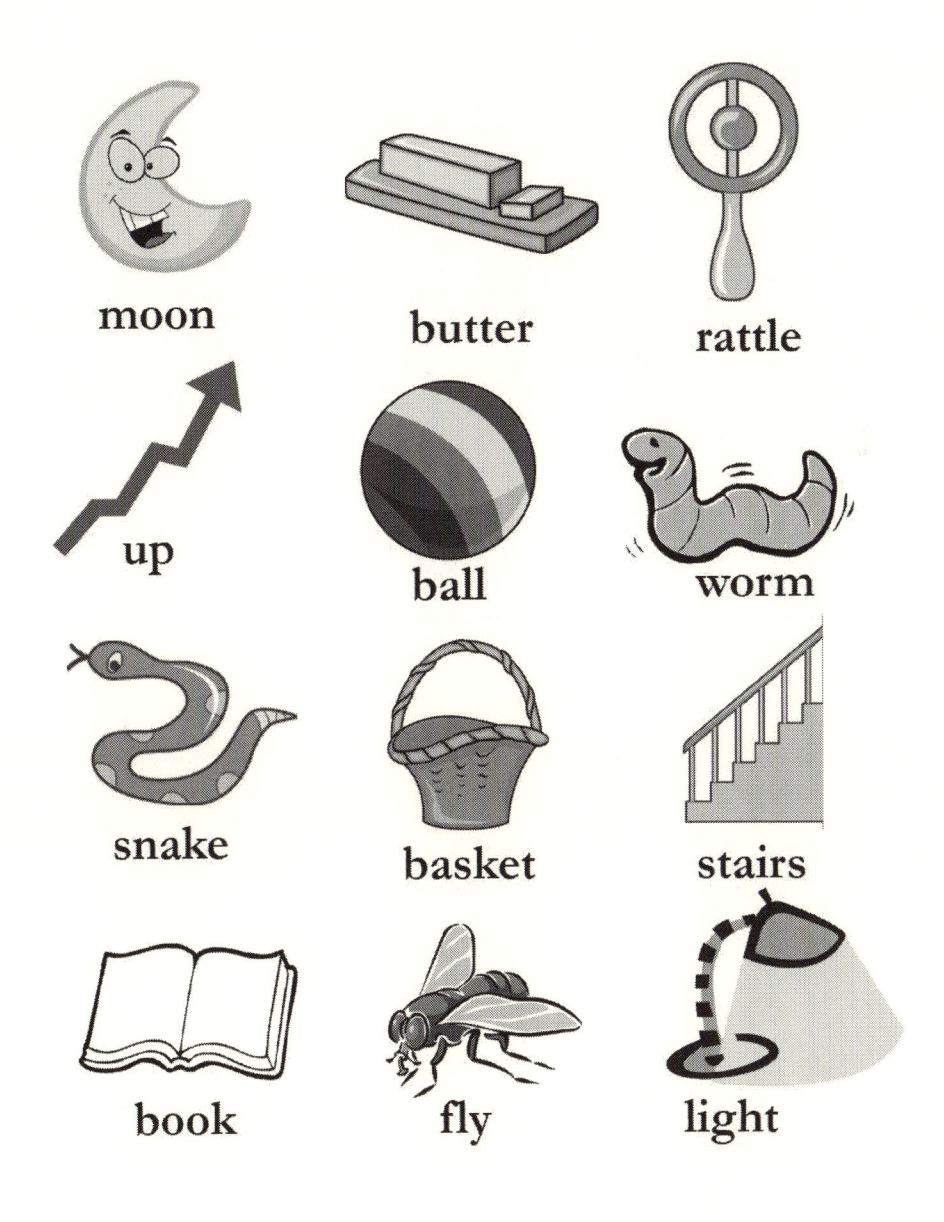

FIND 6 COMPOUND WORDS
(words comprised of 2 smaller words)

moon butter rattle

up ball worm

snake basket stairs

book fly light

ANSWERS TO: FIND 6 COMPOUND WORDS

1. moonlight

2. butterfly

3. rattlesnake

4. upstairs

5. basketball

6. bookworm

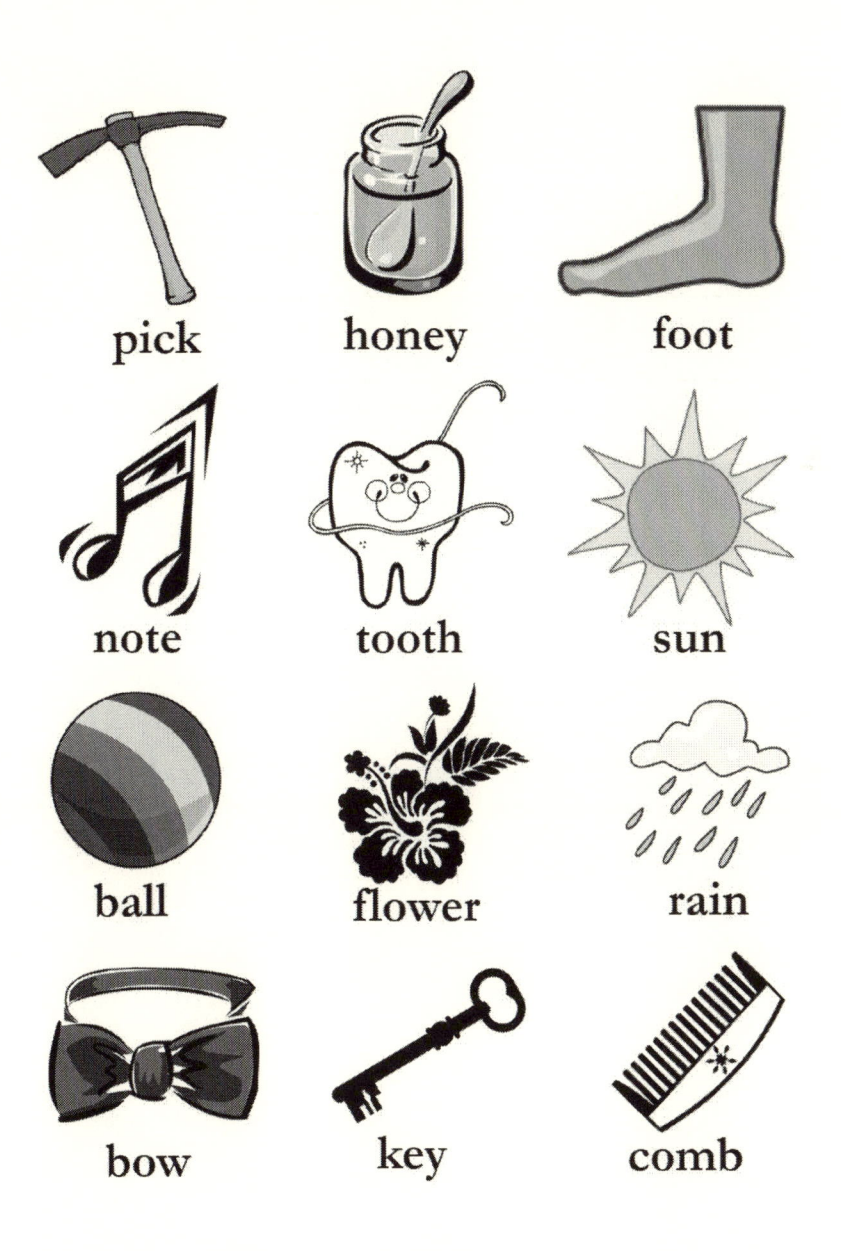

FIND 6 COMPOUND WORDS
(words comprised of 2 smaller words)

pick	honey	foot
note	tooth	sun
ball	flower	rain
bow	key	comb

ANSWERS TO: FIND 6 COMPOUND WORDS

1. _____toothpick_____

2. _____honeycomb_____

3. _____football_____

4. _____keynote_____

5. _____sunflower_____

6. _____rainbow_____

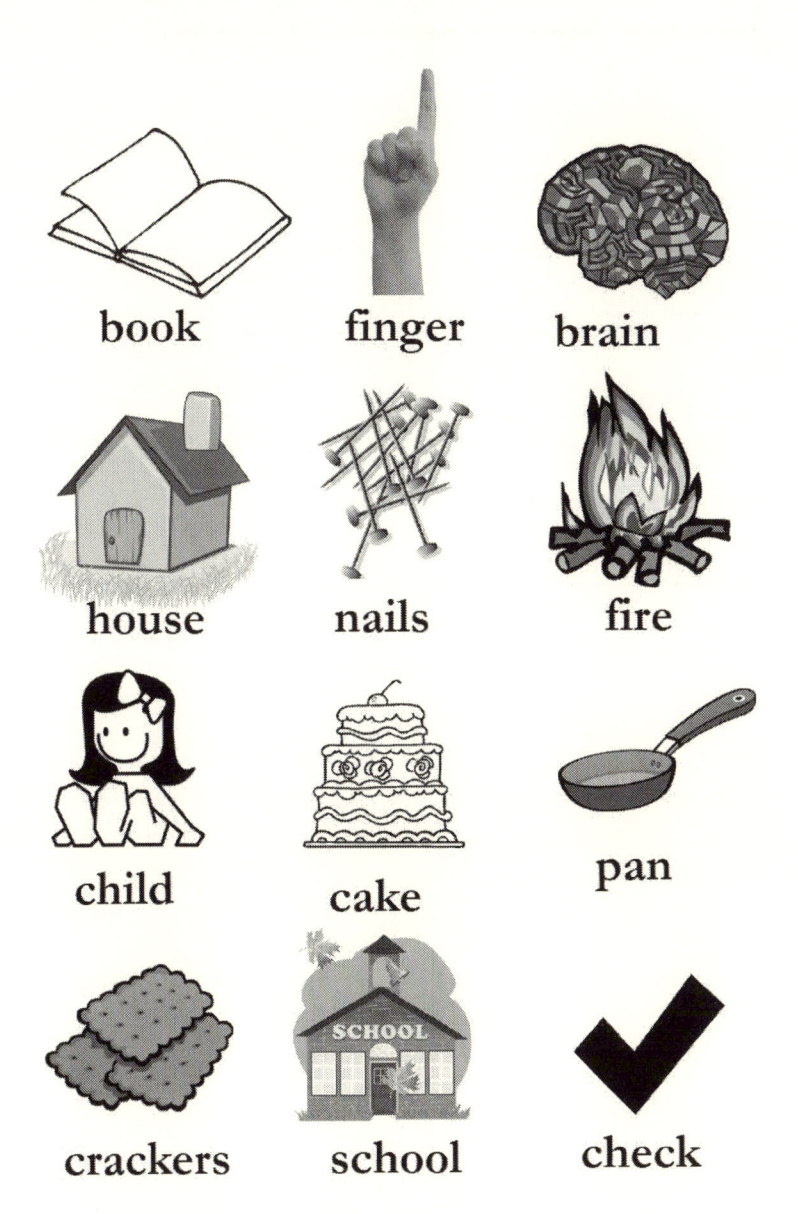

FIND 6 COMPOUND WORDS
(words comprised of 2 smaller words)

book	finger	brain
house	nails	fire
child	cake	pan
crackers	school	check

ANSWERS TO: FIND 6 COMPOUND WORDS

1. checkbook

2. fingernails

3. brainchild

4. schoolhouse

5. firecrackers

6. pancake

FIND 6 COMPOUND WORDS
(words comprised of 2 smaller words)

board	pool	bed
room	arm	water
stripes	card	car
four	melon	pin

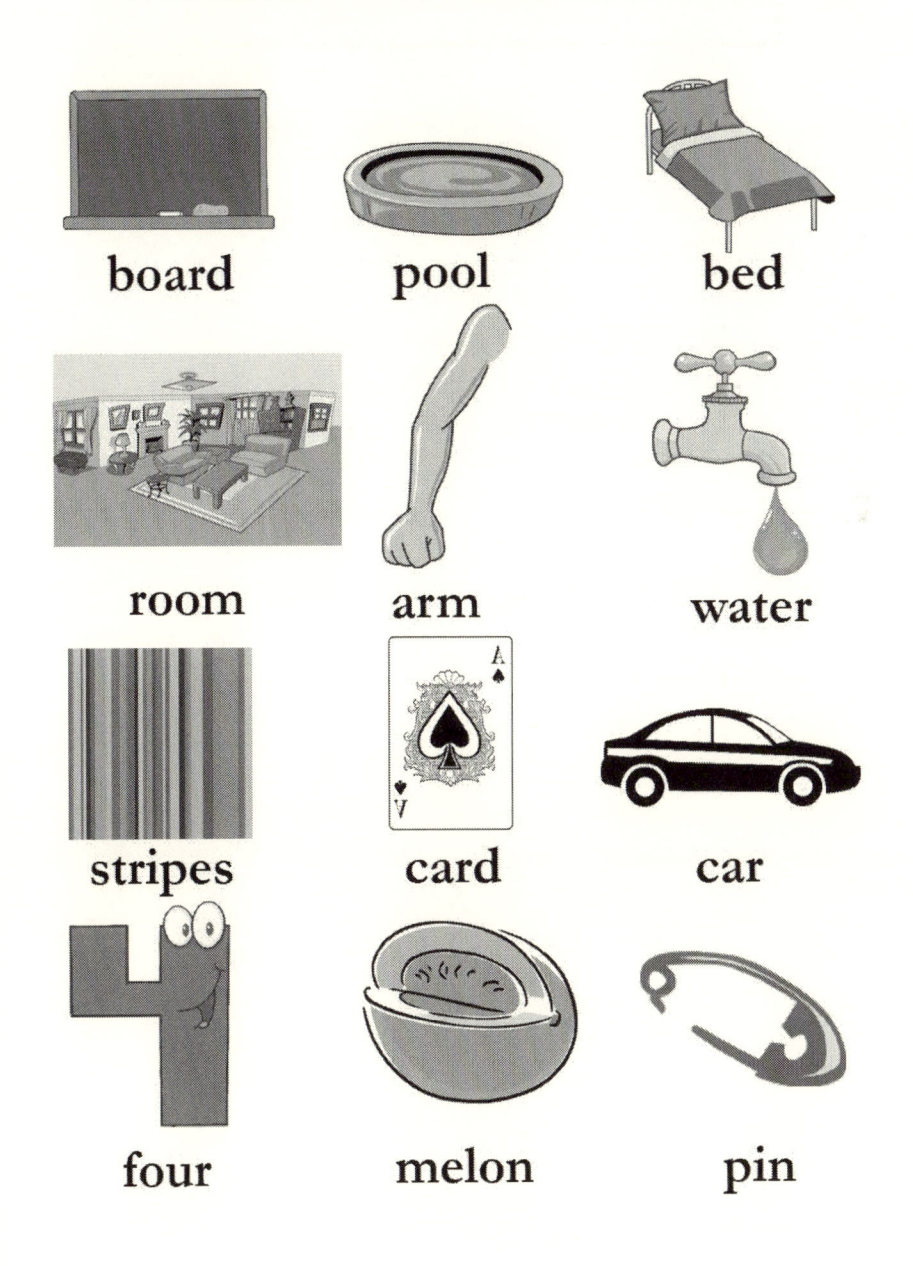

ANSWERS TO: FIND 6 COMPOUND WORDS

1. _____cardboard_____

2. _____carpool_____

3. _____bedroom_____

4. _____forearm_____

5. _____watermelon_____

6. _____pinstripes_____

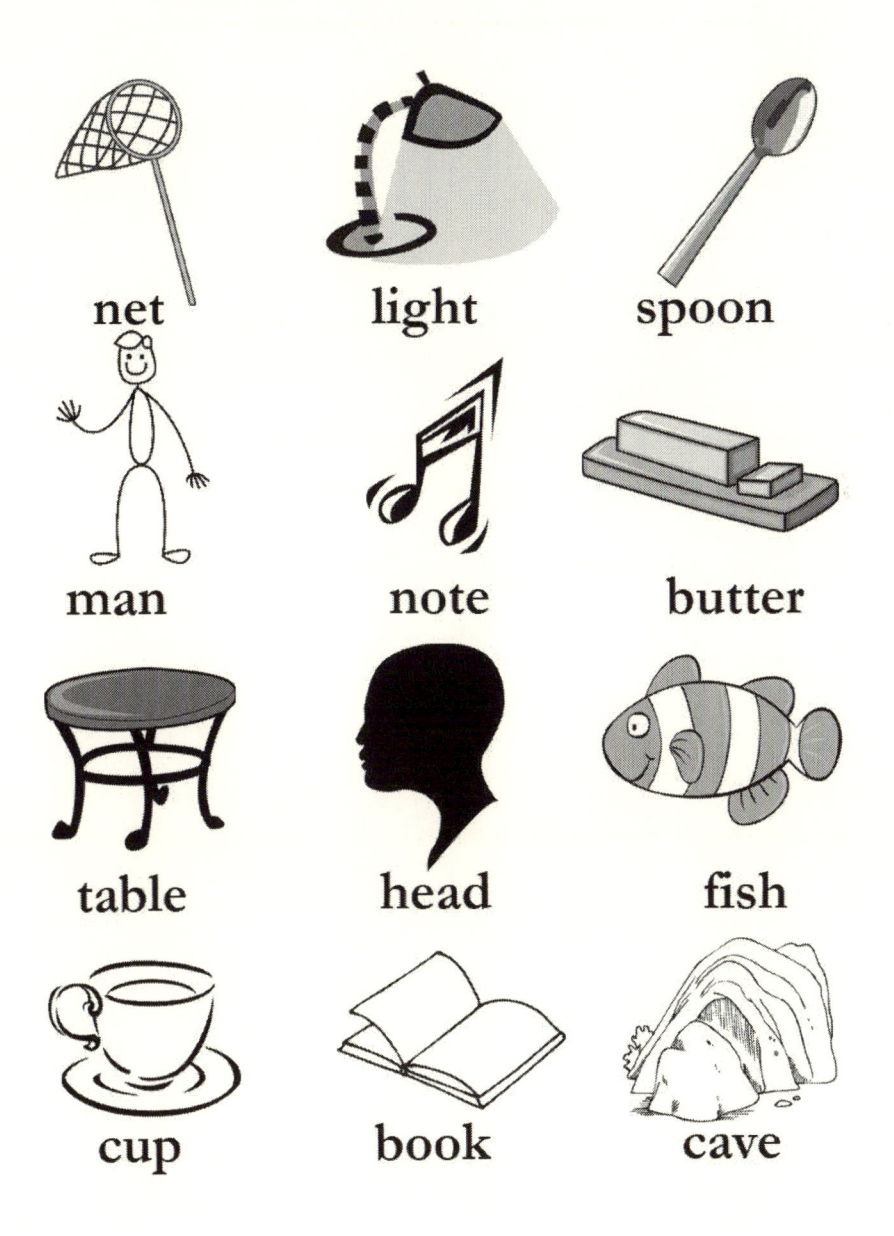

FIND 6 COMPOUND WORDS
(words comprised of 2 smaller words)

net	light	spoon
man	note	butter
table	head	fish
cup	book	cave

ANSWERS TO: FIND 6 COMPOUND WORDS

1. _____fishnet_____

2. _____headlight_____

3. _____tablespoon_____

4. _____caveman_____

5. _____notebook_____

6. _____buttercup_____

APPENDIX

This Appendix includes reproducible "Bingo" game boards that provide an opportunity for group interaction. Each player is given a copy of a game board. The boards contain pictures of words used in Game #2, "Word Pairs—Objects." For example, Boards A1 through A6 have pictures corresponding to word pairs on Page 11; Boards B1 through B6 have pictures representing items on Page 13, and so forth, through Board F6.

The game is played in the same way as classic "Bingo." The "caller" randomly presents questions, and players identify and cross off corresponding pictures on their boards. For example the caller presents a question on Page 11: "Needle goes with _____," and players identify the associated word and picture on Board A1, "thread." Each player whose board contains "thread" crosses it off. The winner is the first person to cover or cross out all pictures on their board.

**Joggin' Your Noggin
Word Pairs
Board A1**

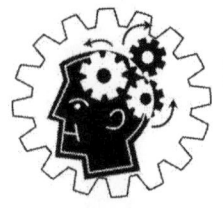

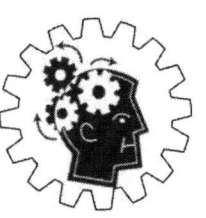

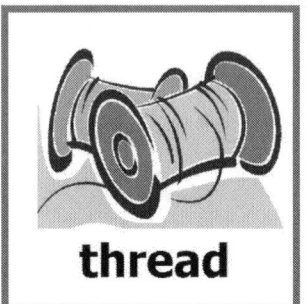

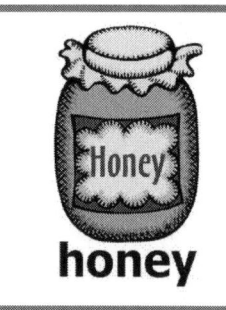

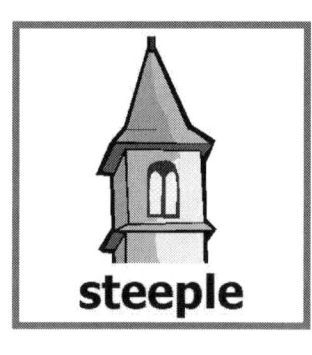

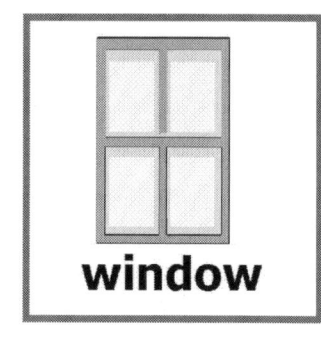

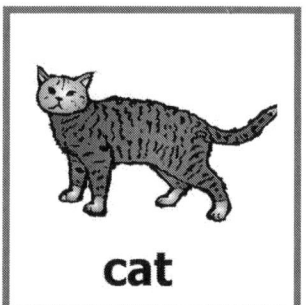

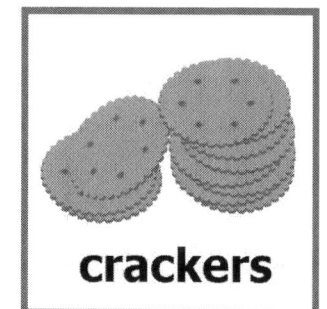

thread

honey

steeple

window

cat

crackers

**Joggin' Your Noggin
Word Pairs
Board A2**

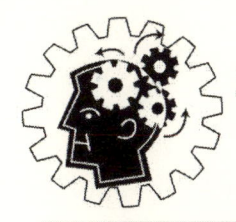

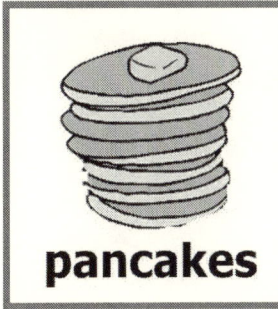

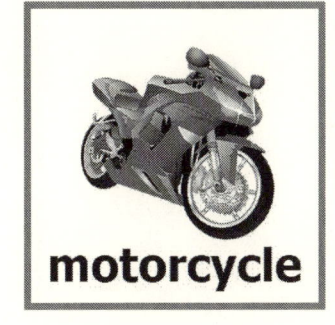

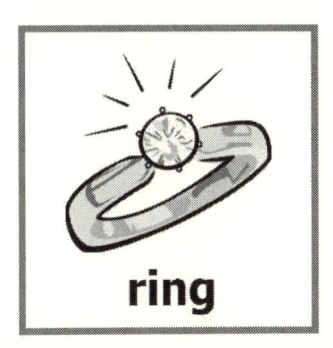

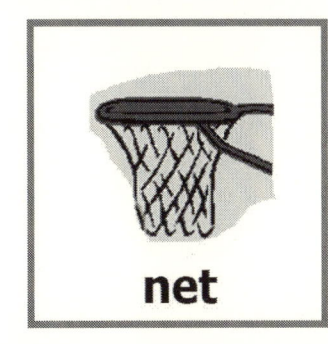

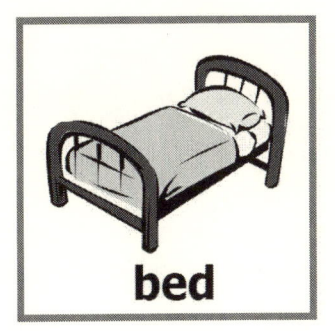

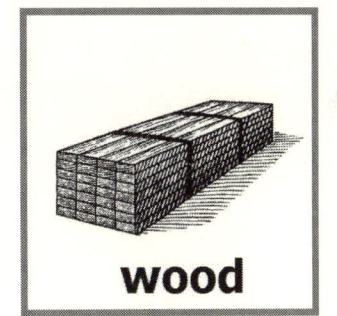

pancakes

motorcycle

ring

net

bed

wood

Joggin' Your Noggin
Word Pairs
Board A3

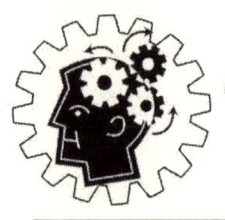

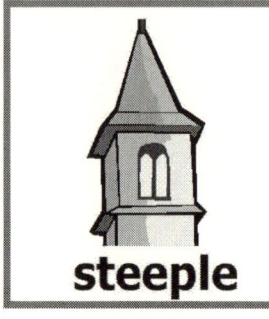

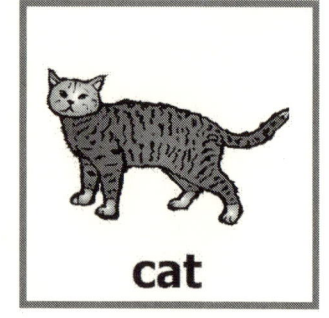

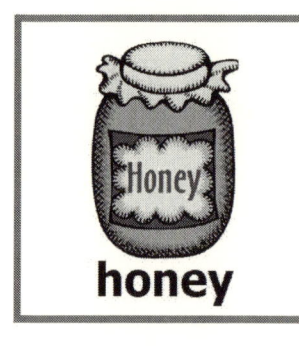

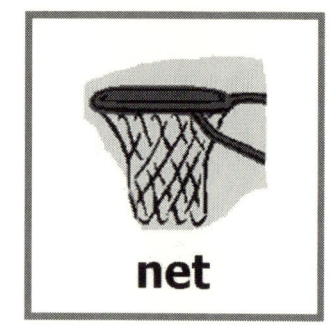

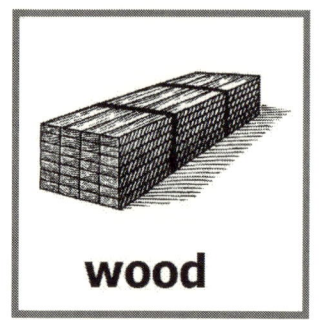

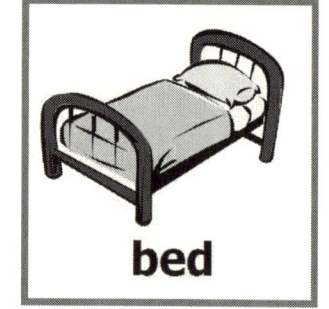

steeple	**cat**
honey	**net**
wood	**bed**

Joggin' Your Noggin
Word Pairs
Board A4

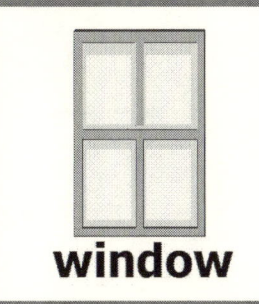

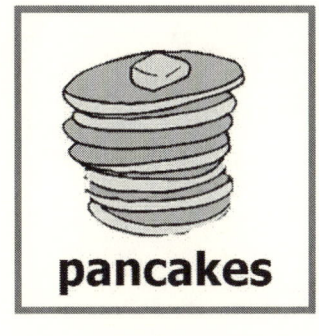

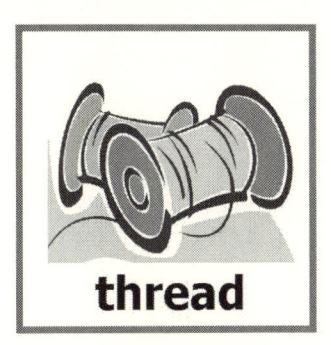

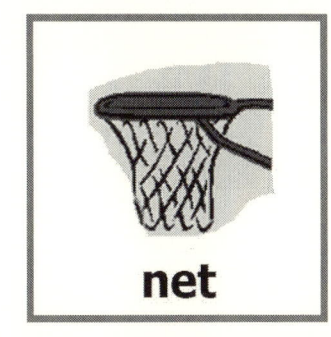

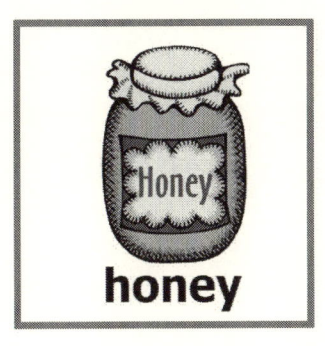

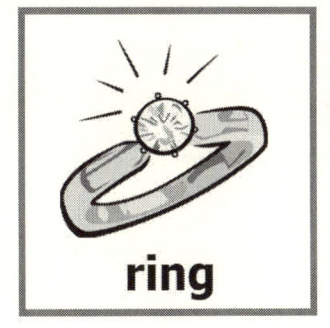

window	pancakes
thread	net
honey	ring

Joggin' Your Noggin
Word Pairs
Board A5

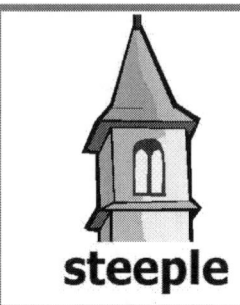

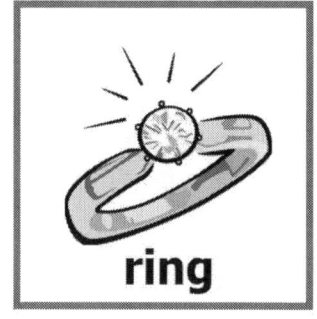

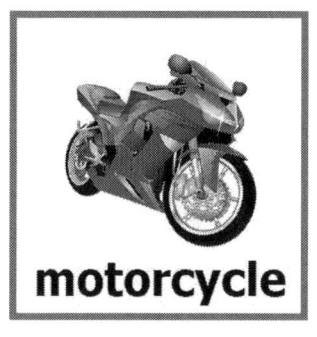

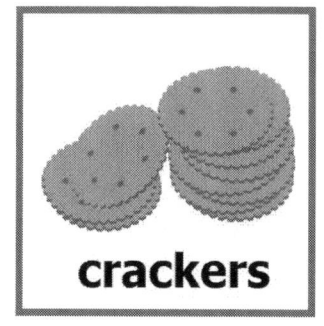

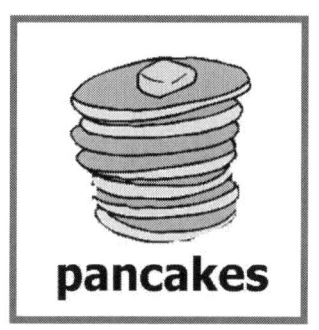

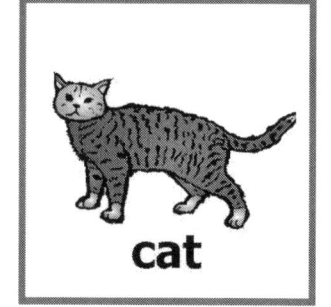

steeple	**ring**
motorcycle	**crackers**
pancakes	**cat**

**Joggin' Your Noggin
Word Pairs
Board A6**

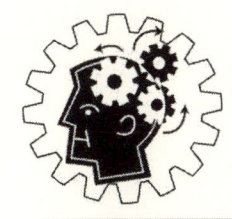

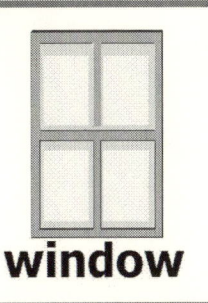

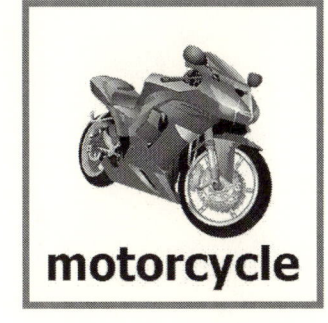

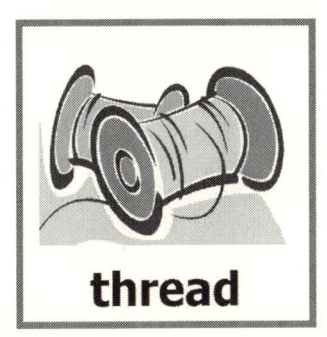

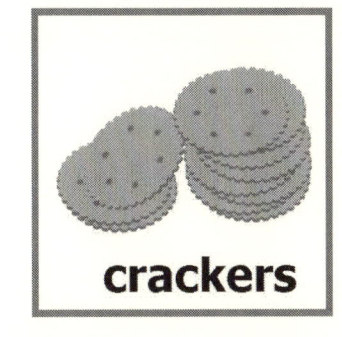

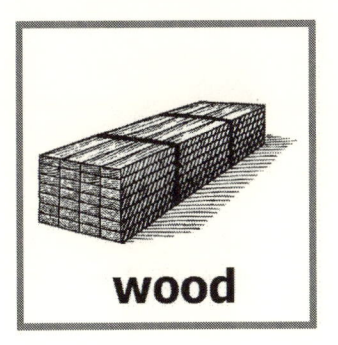

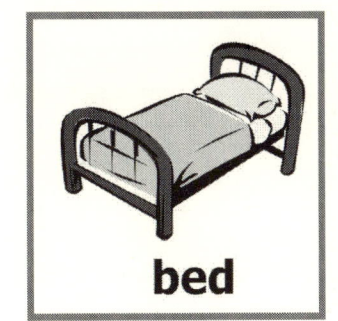

window	motorcycle
thread	crackers
wood	bed

Joggin' Your Noggin
Word Pairs
Board B1

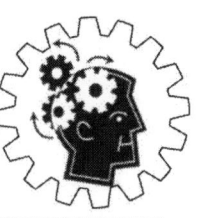

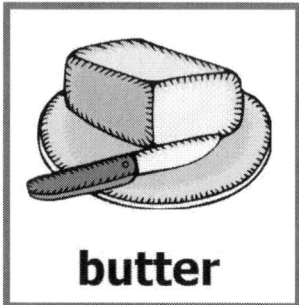

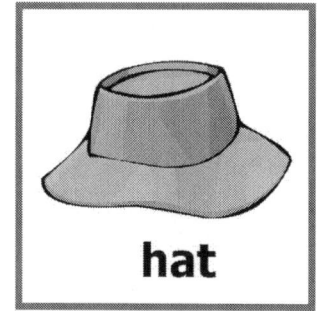

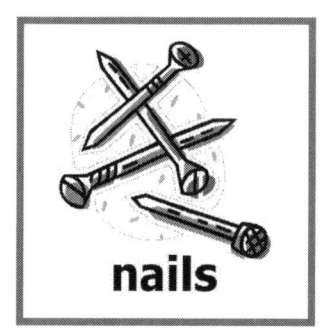

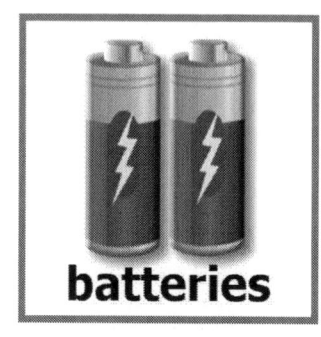

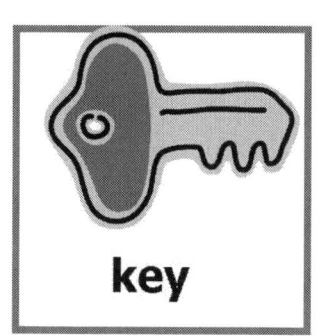

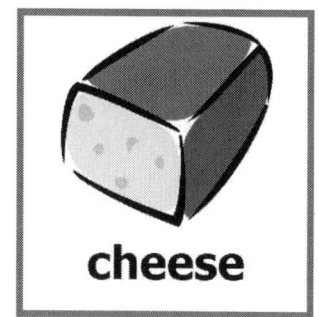

butter

hat

nails

batteries

key

cheese

Joggin' Your Noggin
Word Pairs
Board B2

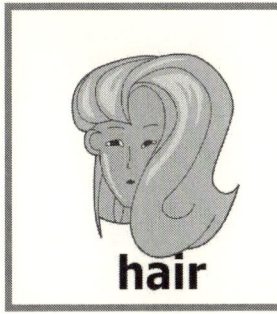

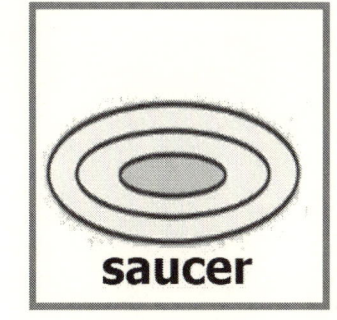

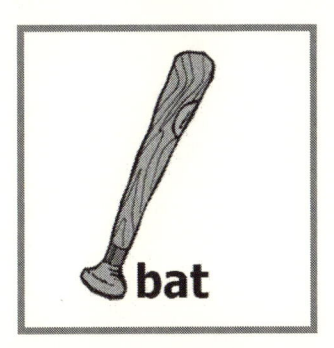

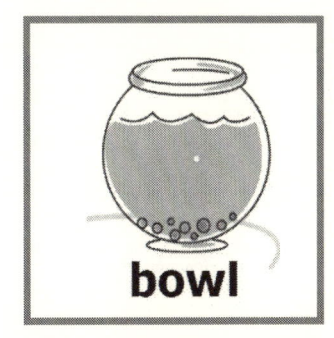

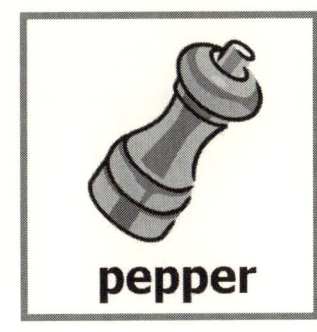

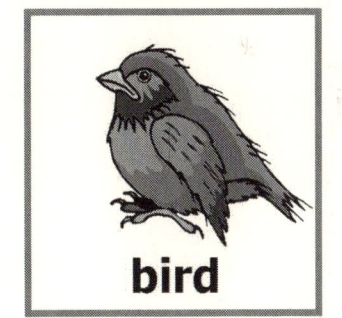

hair	saucer
bat	bowl
pepper	bird

Joggin' Your Noggin
Word Pairs
Board B3

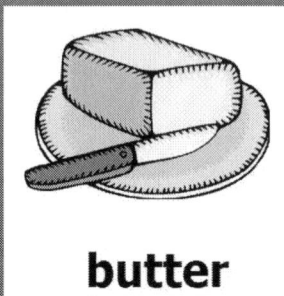

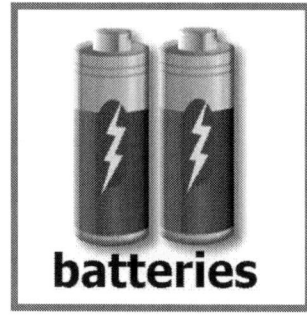

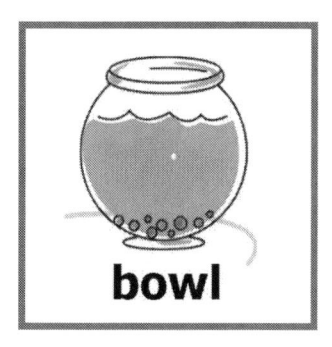

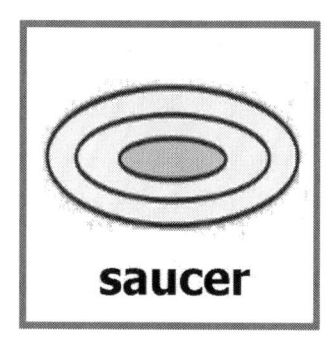

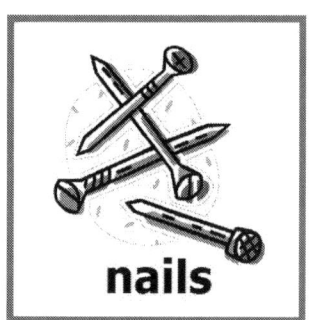

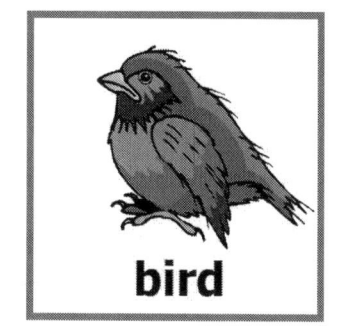

butter	**batteries**
bowl	**saucer**
nails	**bird**

**Joggin' Your Noggin
Word Pairs
Board B4**

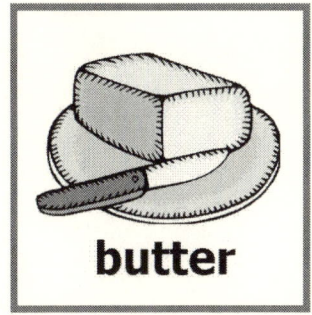

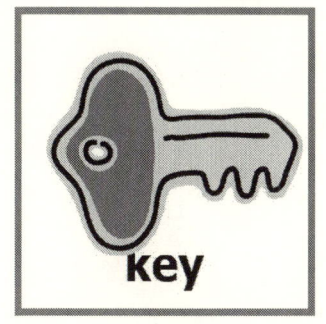

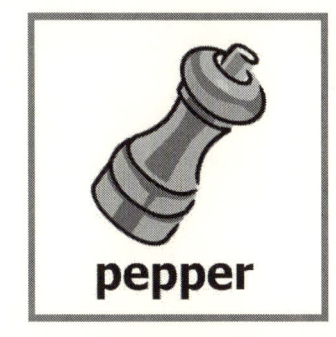

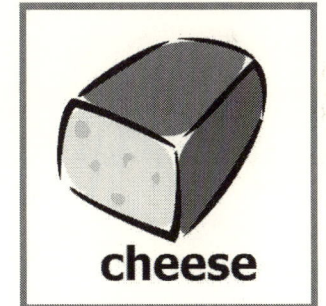

butter

key

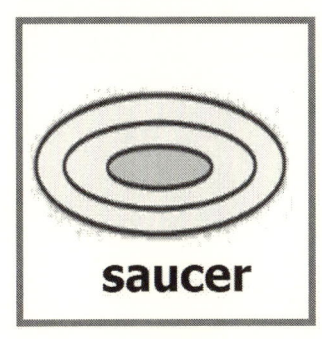

saucer

pepper

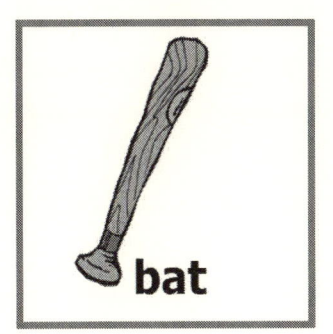

bat

cheese

Joggin' Your Noggin
Word Pairs
Board B5

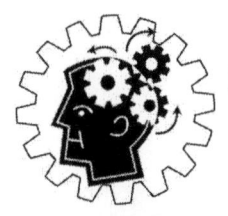

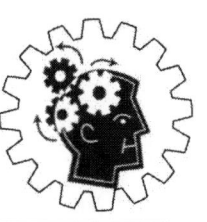

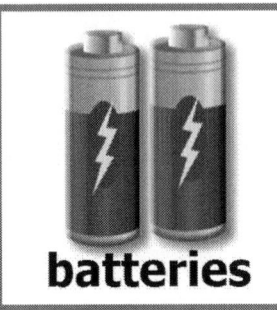

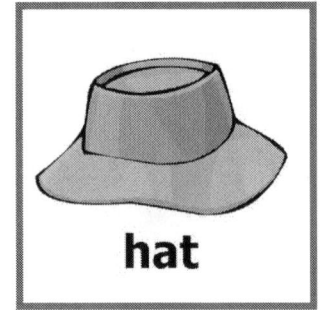

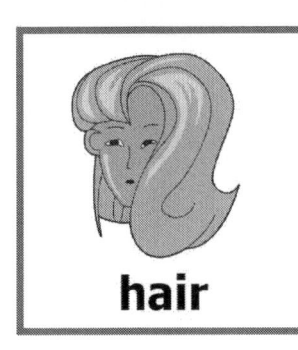

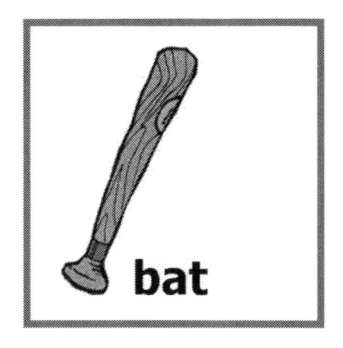

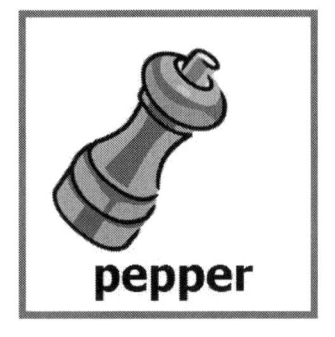

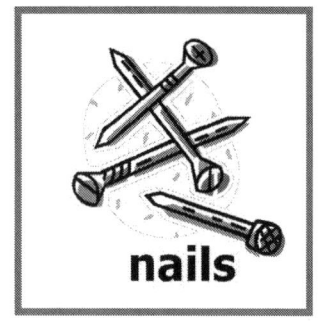

batteries

hat

hair

bat

pepper

nails

Joggin' Your Noggin
Word Pairs
Board B6

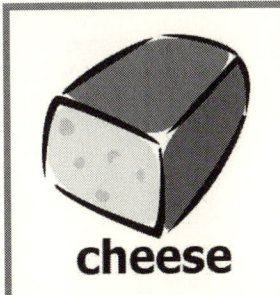

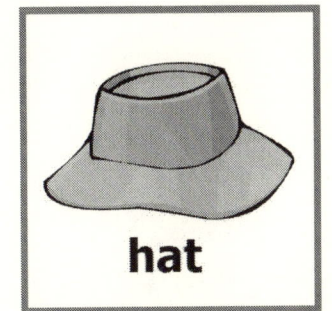

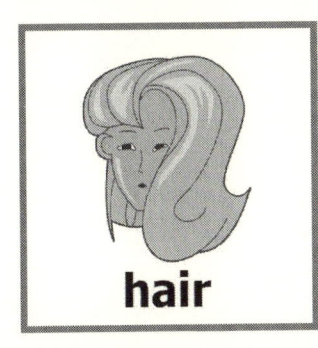

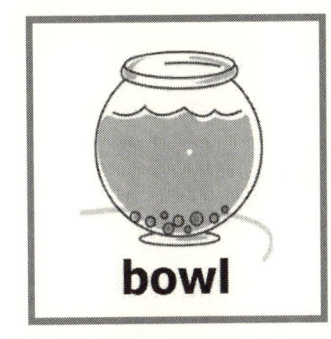

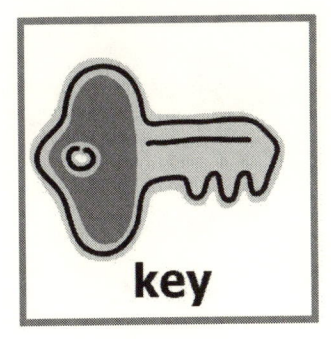

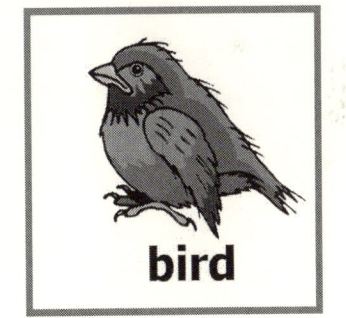

cheese	hat
hair	bowl
key	bird

Joggin' Your Noggin
Word Pairs
Board C1

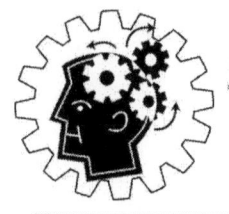

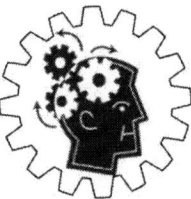

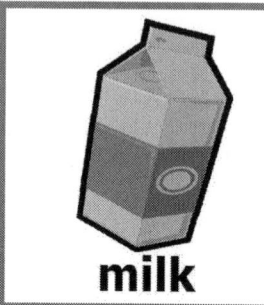

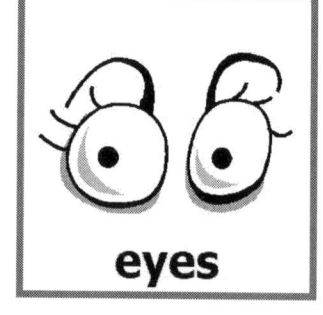

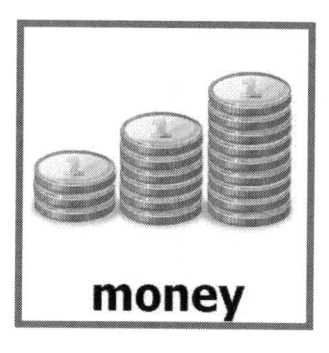

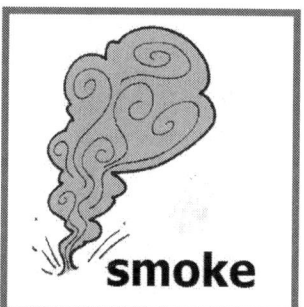

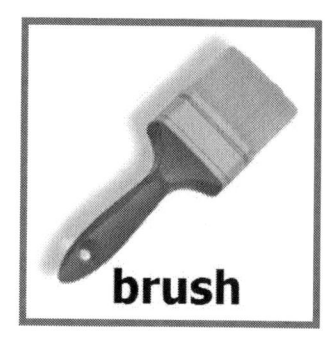

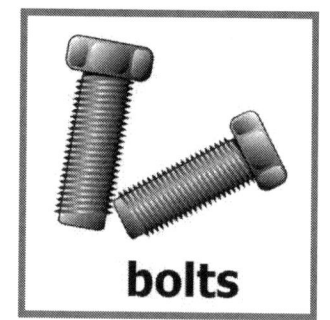

milk	eyes
money	brush
smoke	bolts

Joggin' Your Noggin
Word Pairs
Board C2

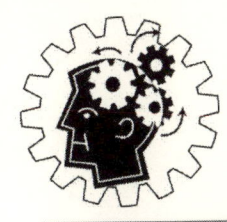

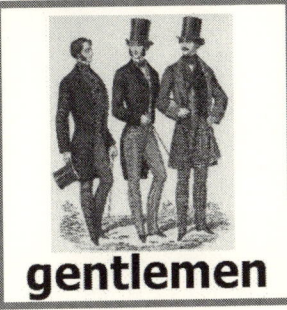

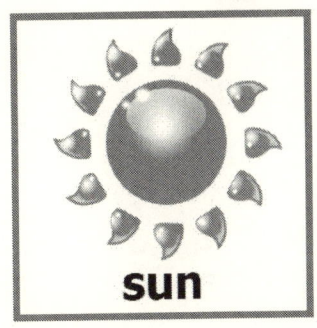

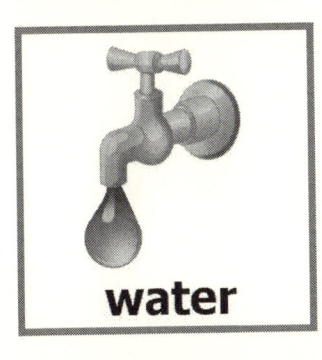

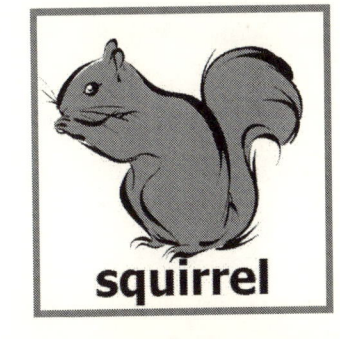

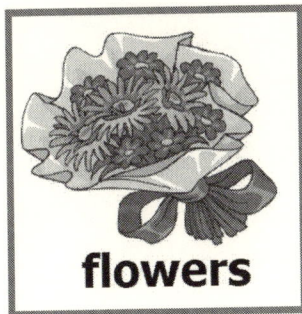

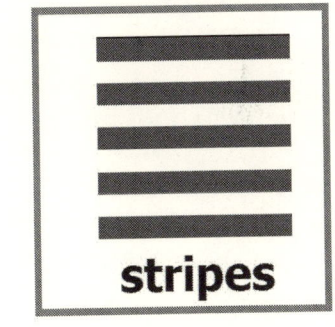

gentlemen	**sun**
water	**squirrel**
flowers	**stripes**

Joggin' Your Noggin
Word Pairs
Board C3

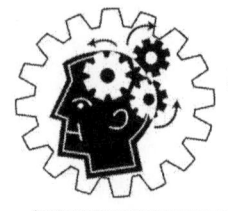

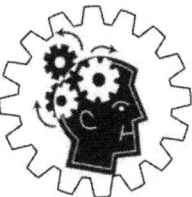

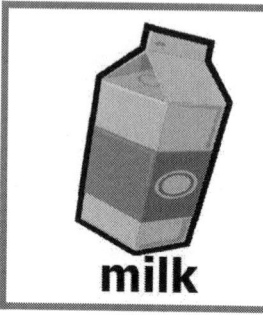

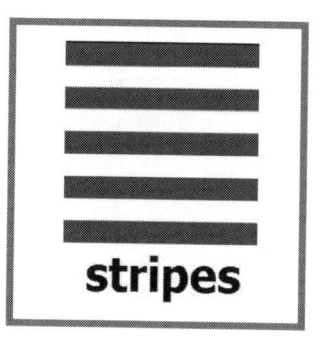

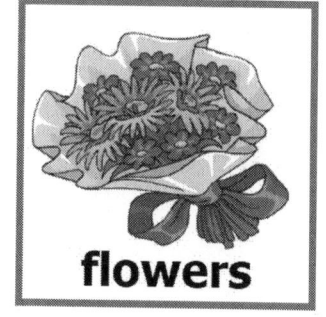

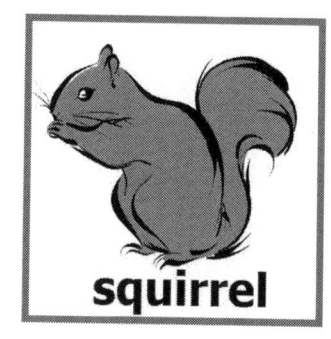

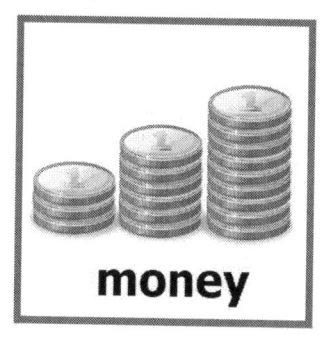

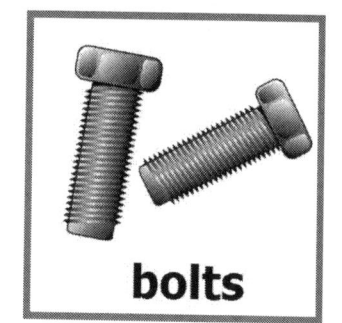

milk	flowers
stripes	squirrel
money	bolts

**Joggin' Your Noggin
Word Pairs
Board C4**

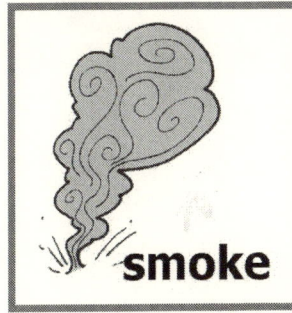

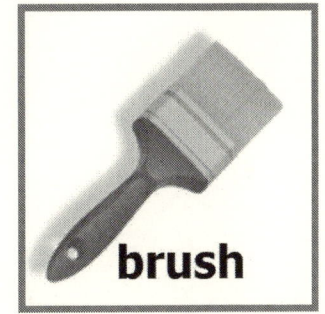

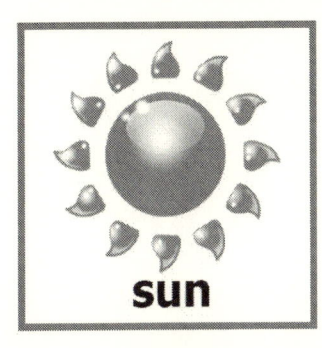

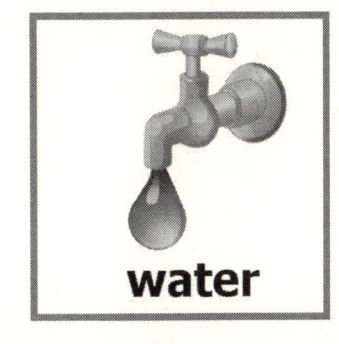

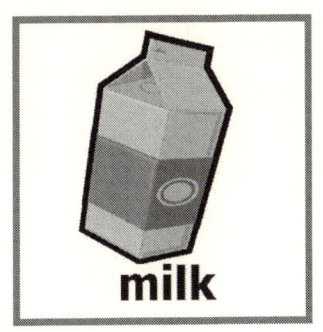

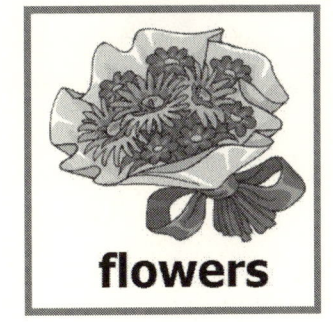

smoke	brush
sun	water
milk	flowers

Joggin' Your Noggin
Word Pairs
Board C5

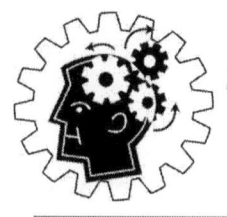

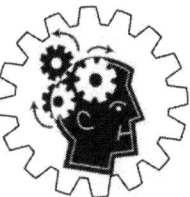

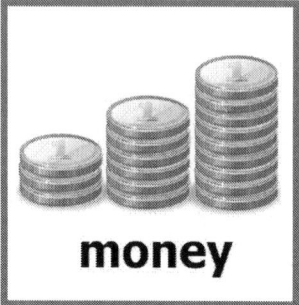

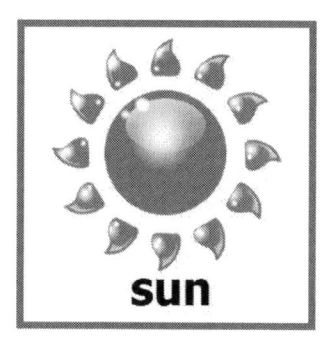

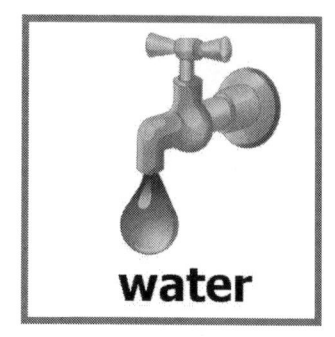

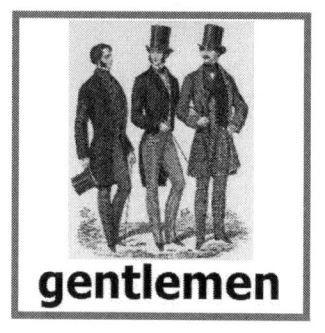

money

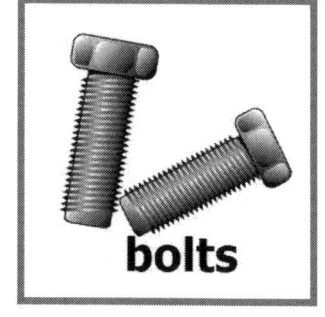

bolts

sun

water

gentlemen

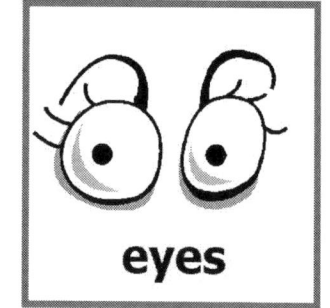

eyes

**Joggin' Your Noggin
Word Pairs
Board C6**

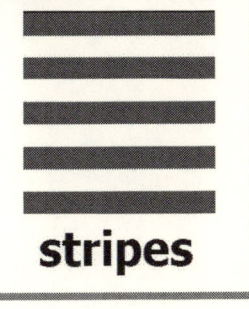

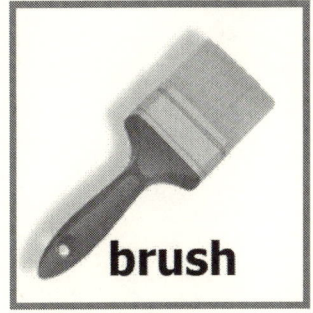

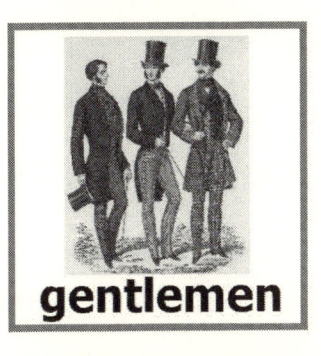

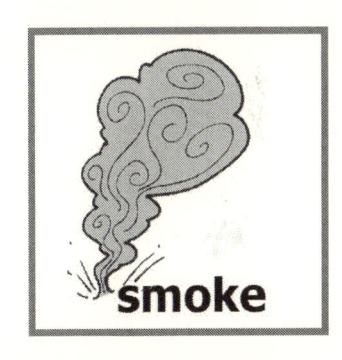

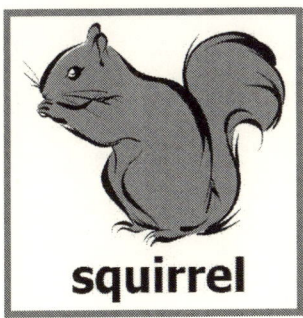

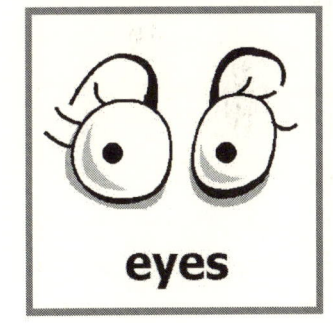

stripes

brush

gentlemen

smoke

squirrel

eyes

Joggin' Your Noggin
Word Pairs
Board D1

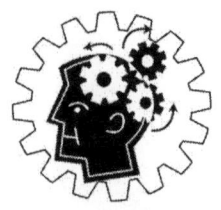

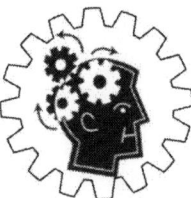

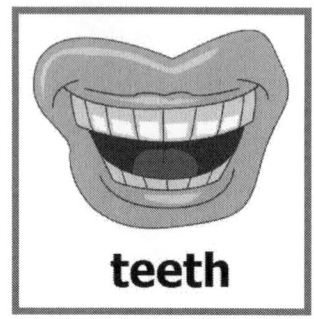

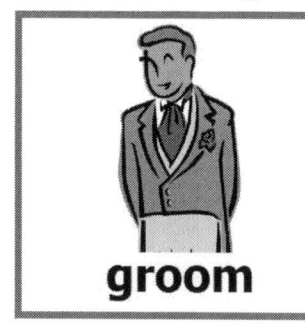

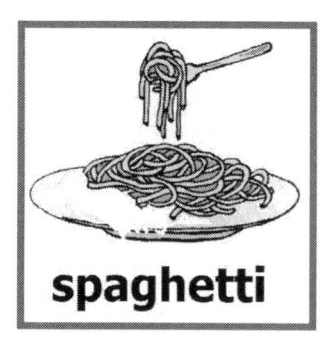

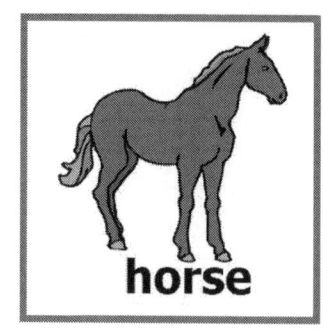

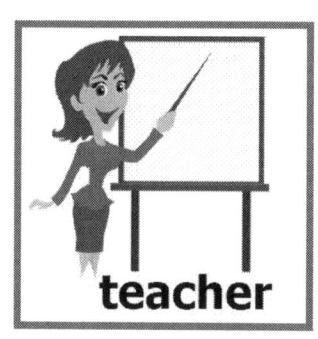

teeth

groom

spaghetti

horse

teacher

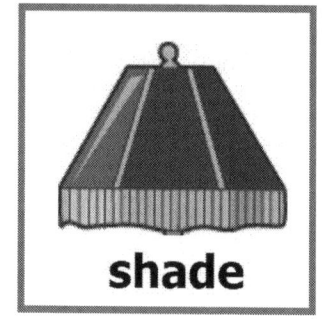

shade

**Joggin' Your Noggin
Word Pairs
Board D2**

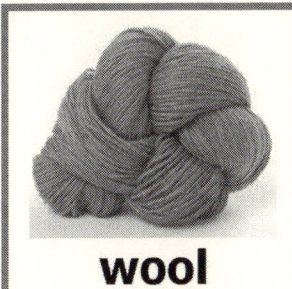

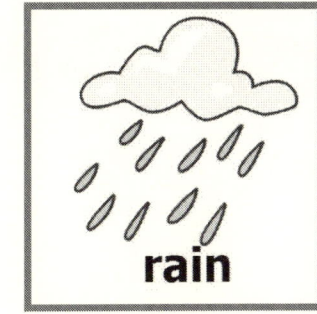

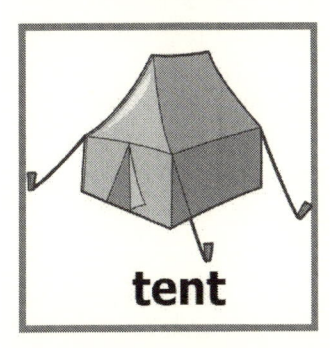

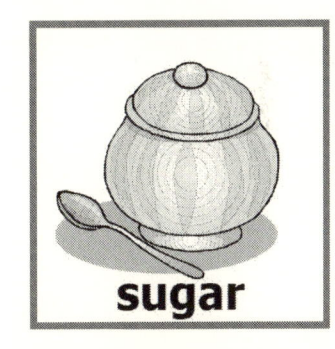

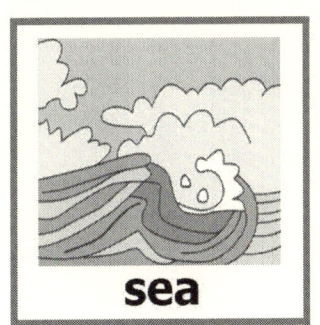

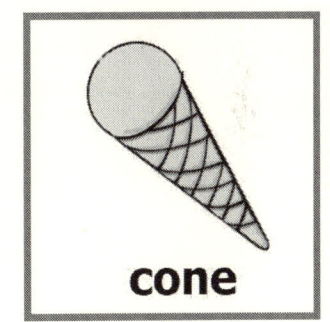

wool

rain

tent

sugar

sea

cone

Joggin' Your Noggin
Word Pairs
Board D3

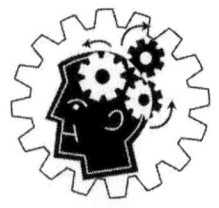

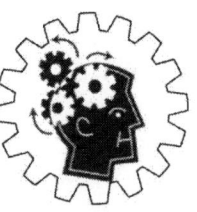

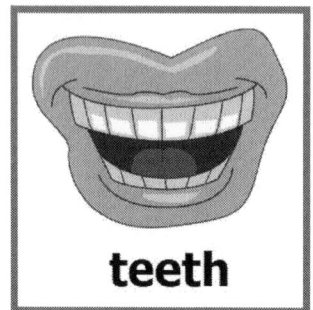

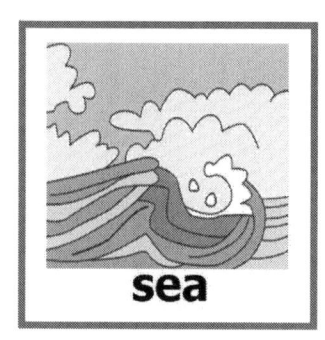

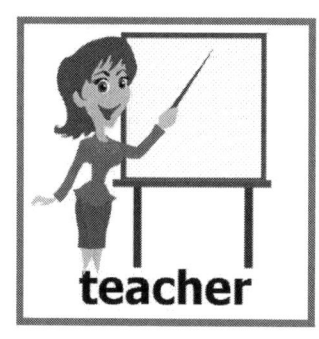

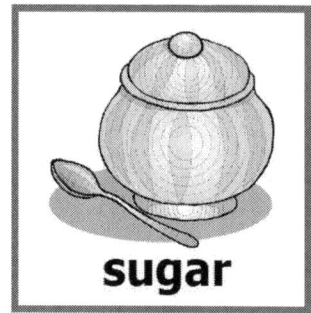

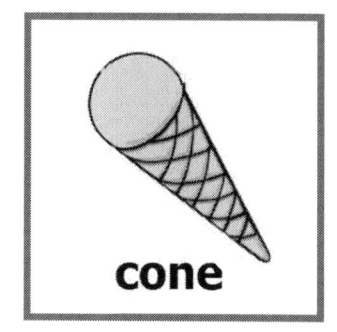

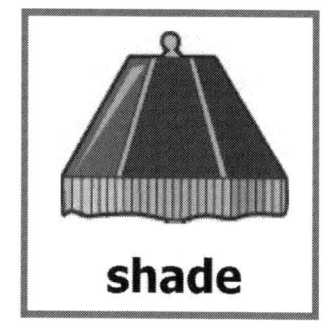

teeth	sugar
sea	cone
teacher	shade

Joggin' Your Noggin
Word Pairs
Board D4

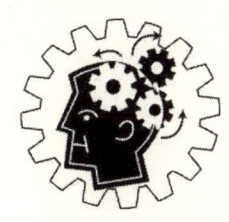

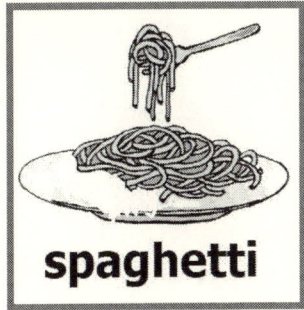

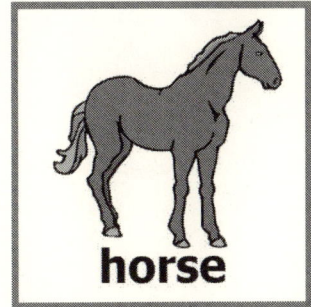

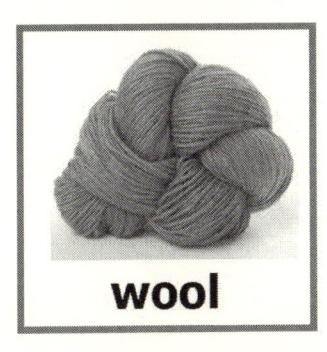

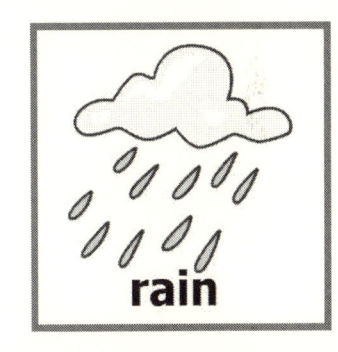

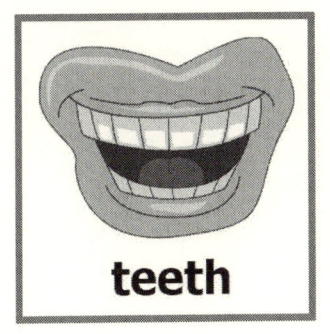

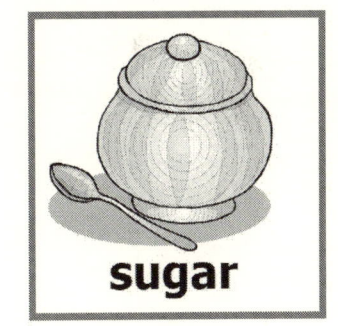

spaghetti	horse
wool	rain
teeth	sugar

Joggin' Your Noggin
Word Pairs
Board D5

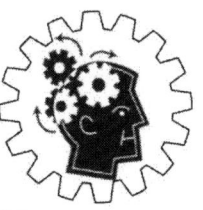

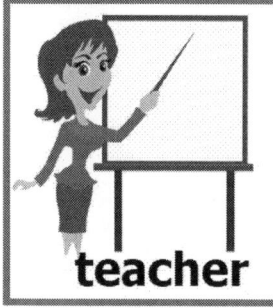

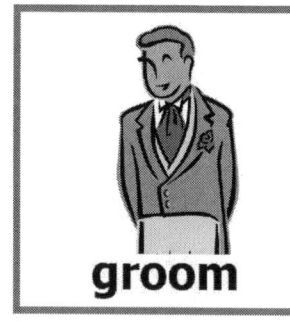

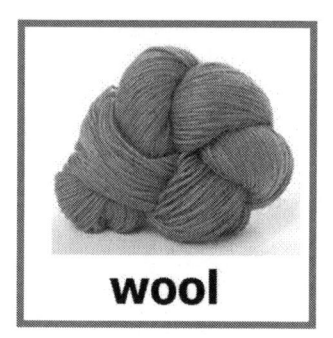

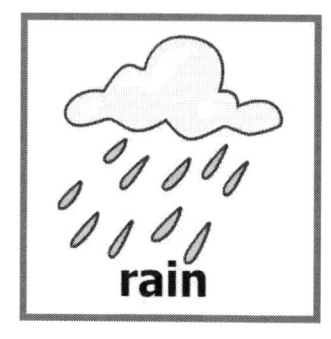

teacher

groom

wool

rain

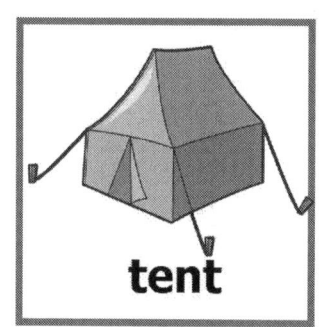

tent

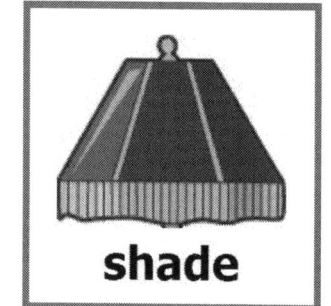

shade

Joggin' Your Noggin
Word Pairs
Board D6

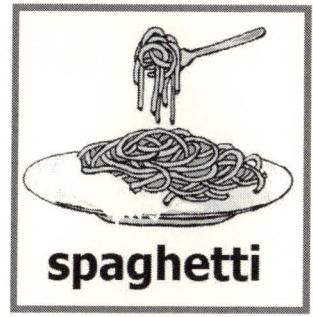

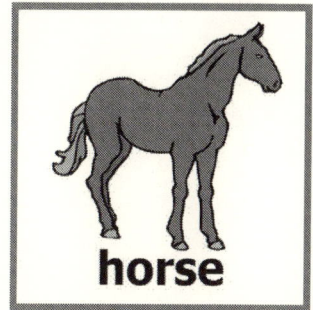

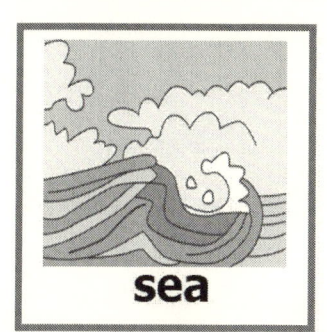

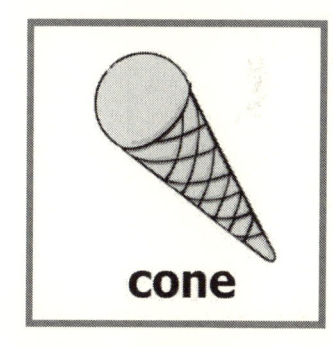

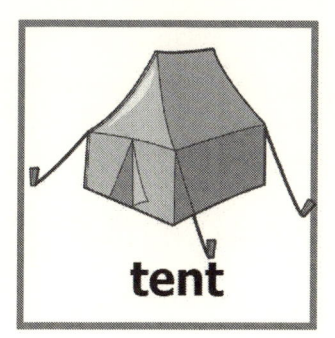

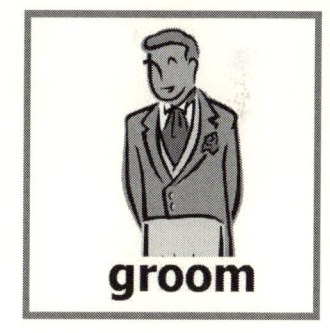

spaghetti	**horse**
sea	**cone**
tent	**groom**

Joggin' Your Noggin
Word Pairs
Board E1

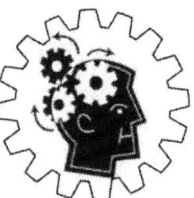

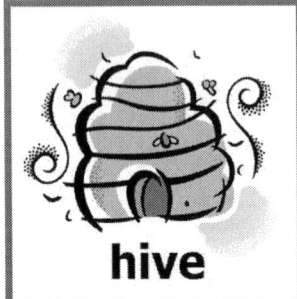

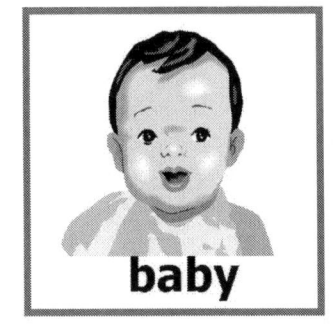

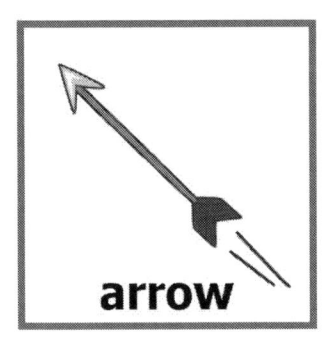

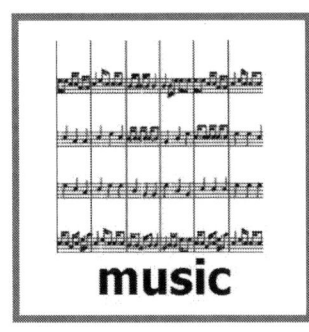

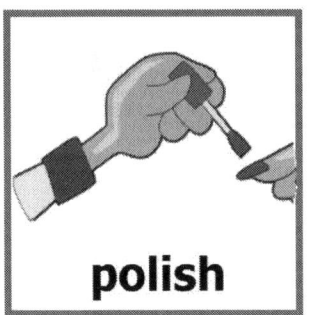

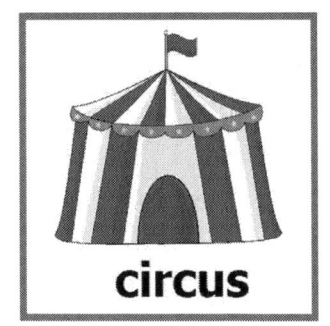

- hive
- baby
- arrow
- music
- polish
- circus

Joggin' Your Noggin
Word Pairs
Board E2

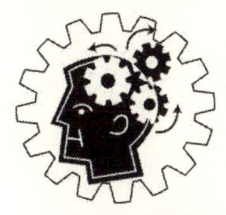

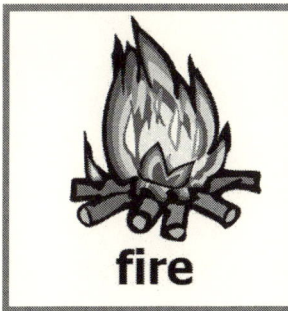

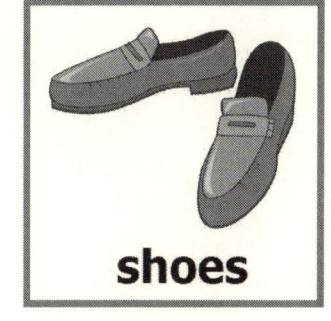

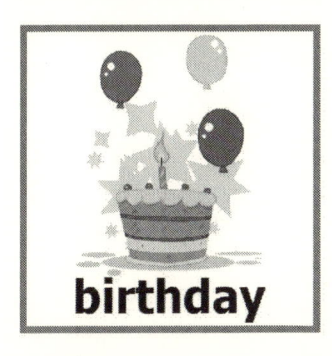

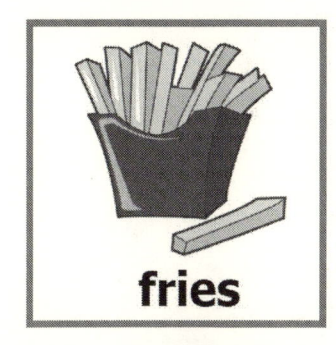

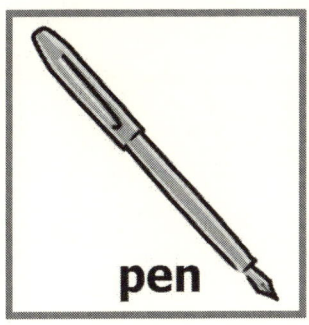

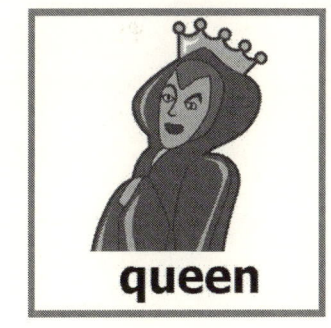

fire	shoes
birthday	fries
pen	queen

Joggin' Your Noggin
Word Pairs
Board E3

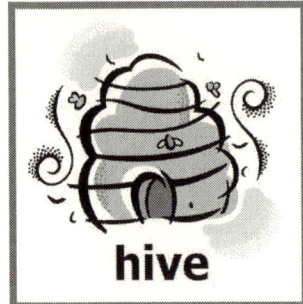

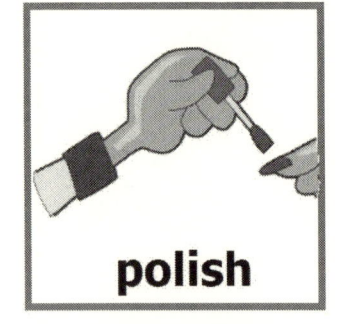

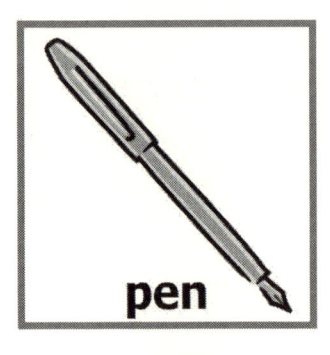

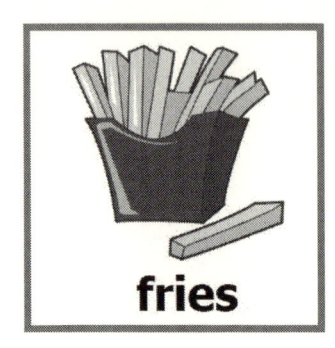

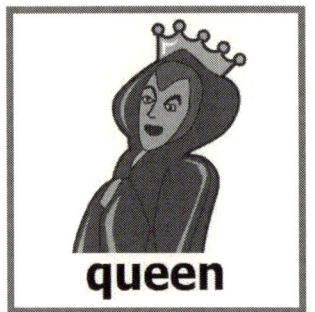

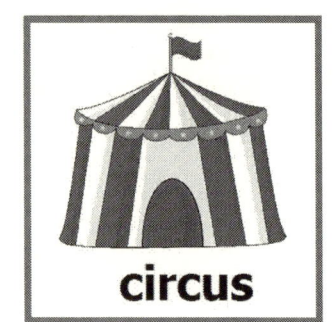

hive

polish

pen

fries

queen

circus

Joggin' Your Noggin
Word Pairs
Board E4

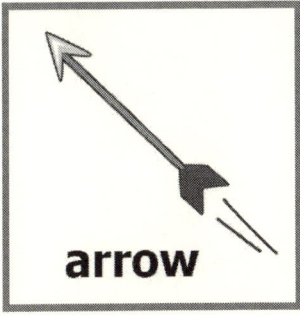

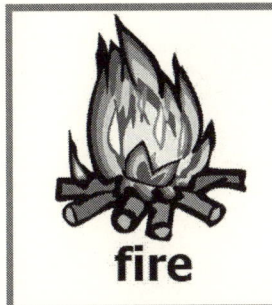

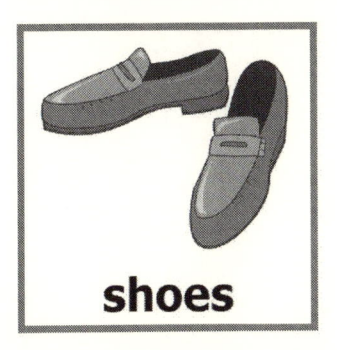

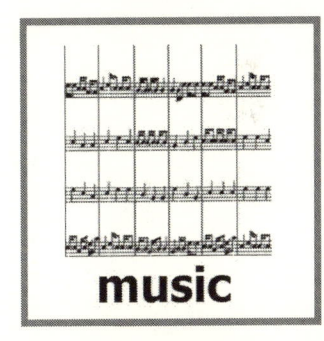

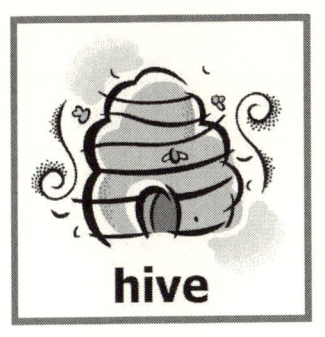

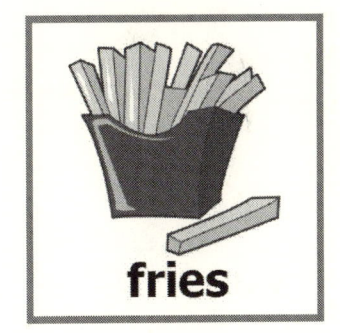

arrow	fire
shoes	music
hive	fries

Joggin' Your Noggin
Word Pairs
Board E5

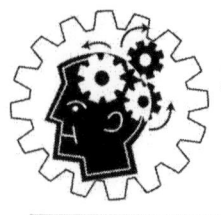

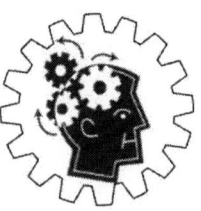

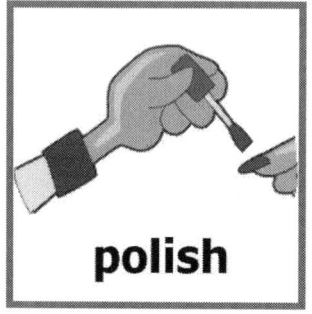

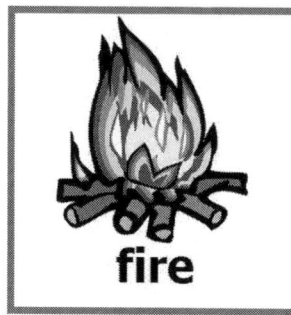

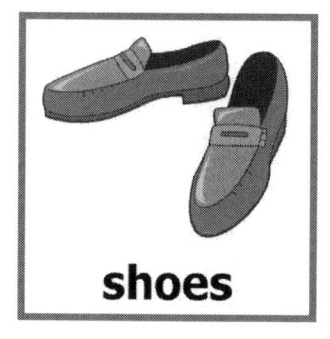

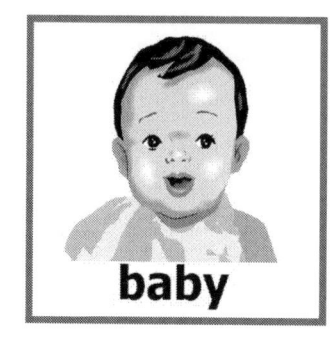

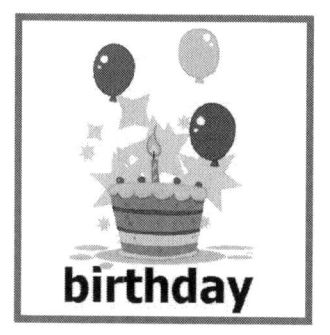

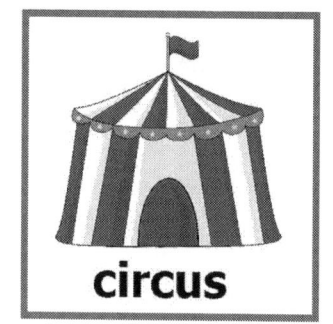

polish

fire

shoes

baby

birthday

circus

Joggin' Your Noggin
Word Pairs
Board E6

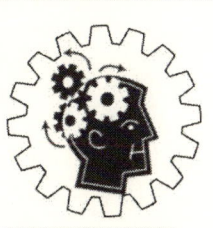

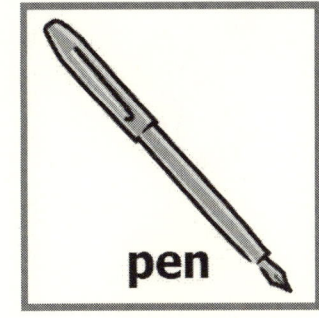

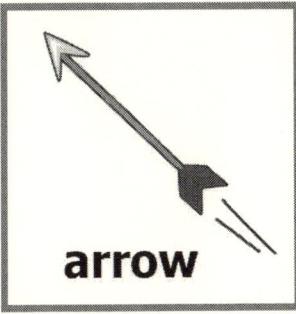

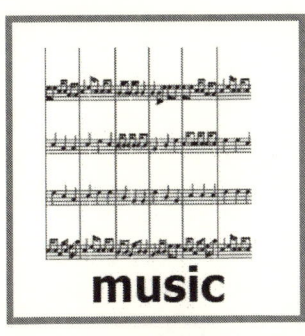

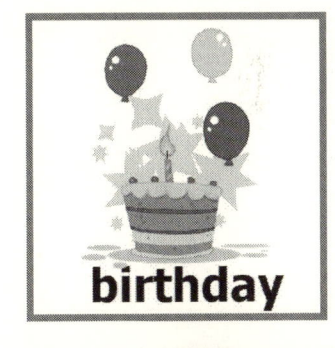

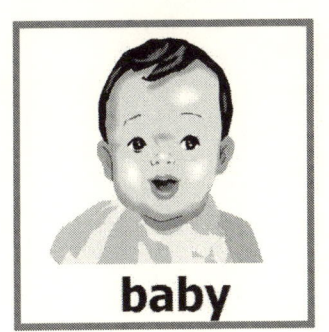

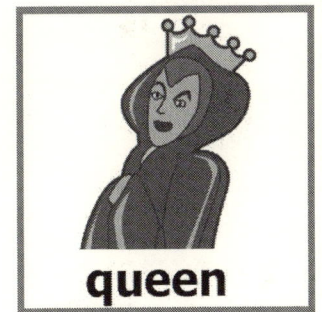

arrow	pen
music	birthday
baby	queen

Joggin' Your Noggin
Word Pairs
Board F1

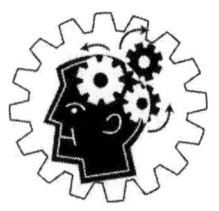

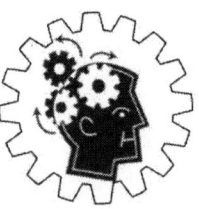

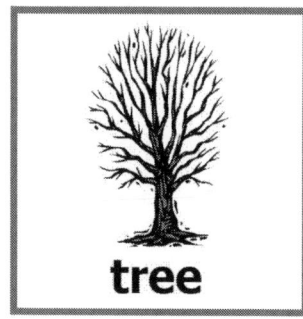

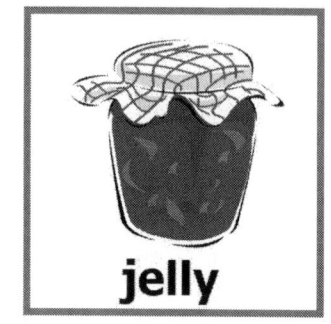

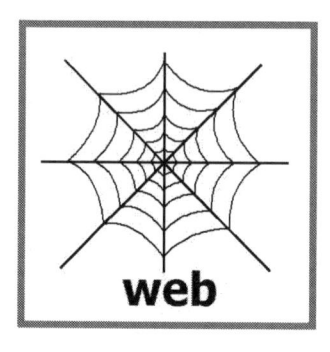

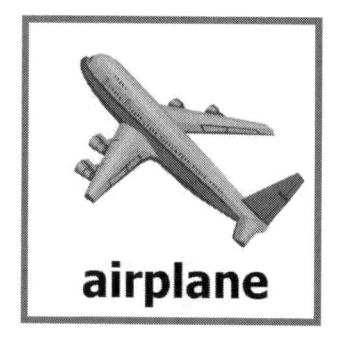

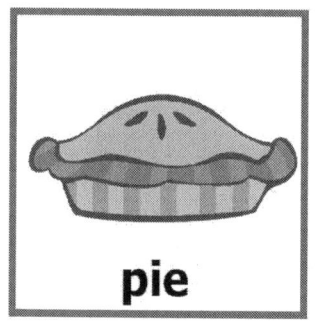

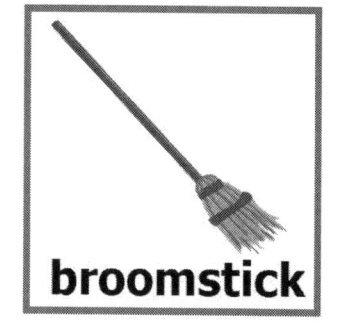

tree	jelly
web	airplane
pie	broomstick

**Joggin' Your Noggin
Word Pairs
Board F2**

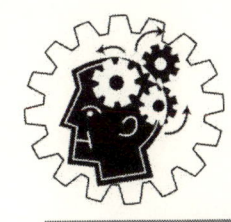

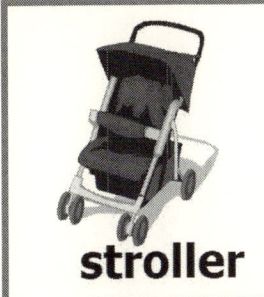

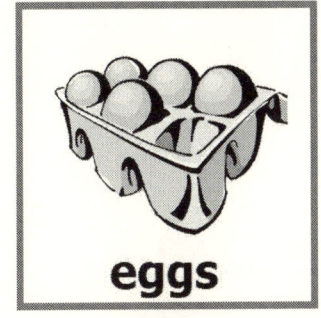

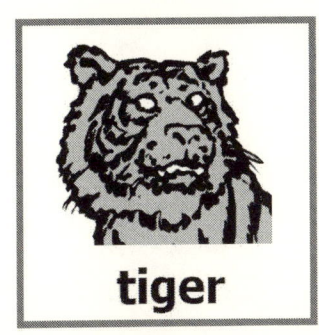

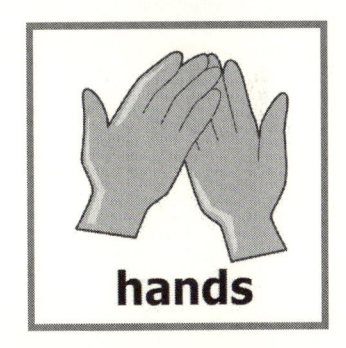

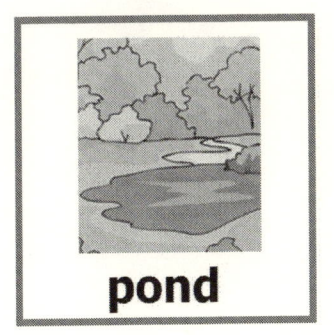

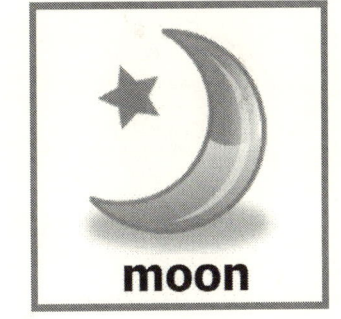

stroller

eggs

tiger

hands

pond

moon

Joggin' Your Noggin
Word Pairs
Board F3

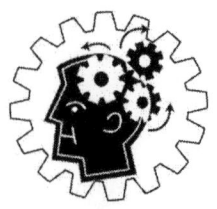

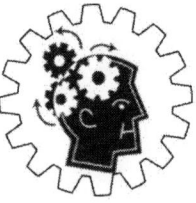

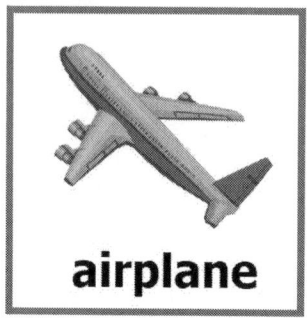

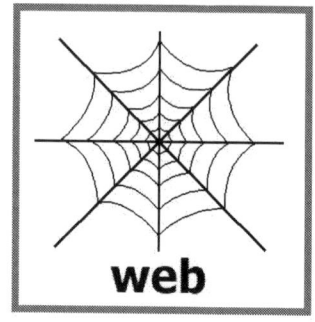

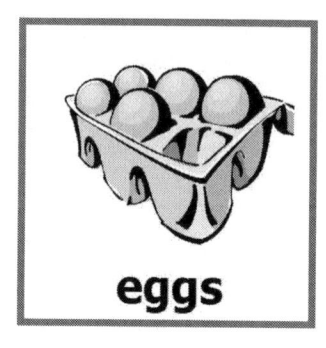

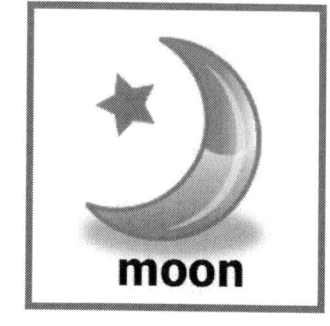

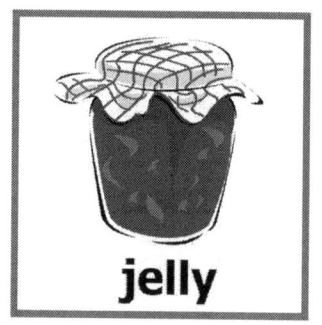

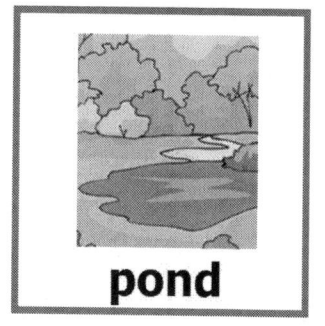

airplane	web
eggs	moon
jelly	pond

**Joggin' Your Noggin
Word Pairs
Board F4**

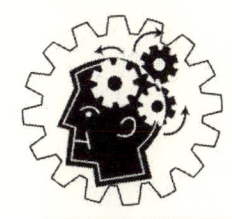

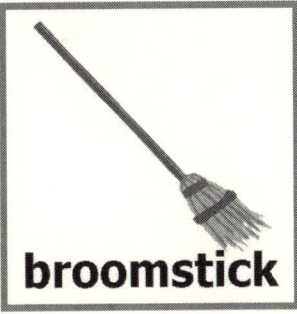

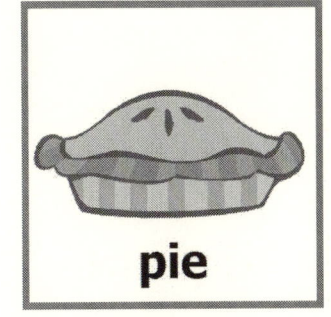

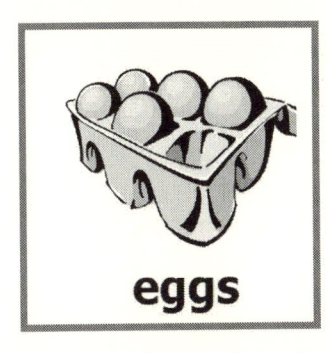

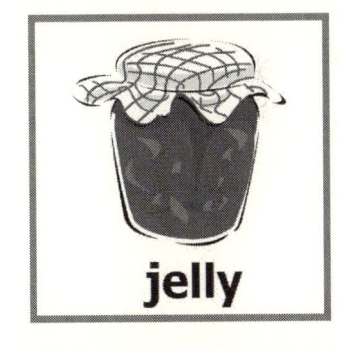

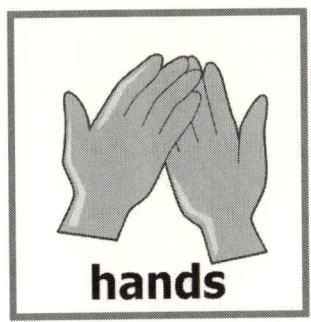

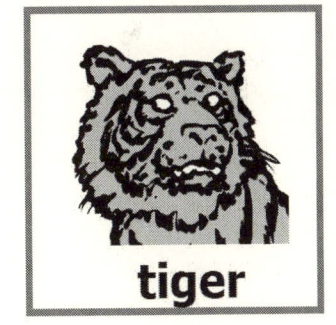

broomstick	pie
eggs	jelly
hands	tiger

**Joggin' Your Noggin
Word Pairs
Board F5**

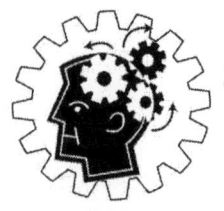

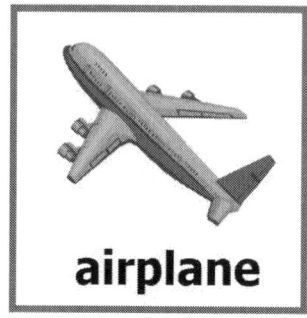

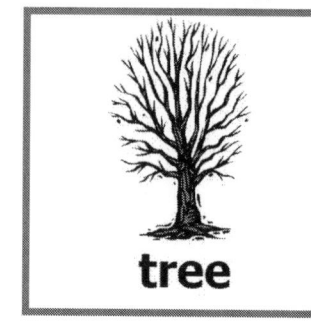

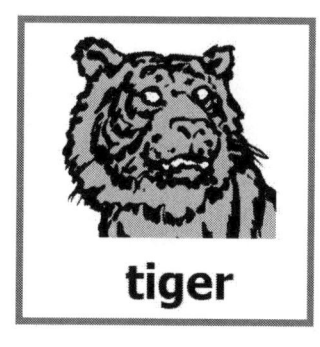

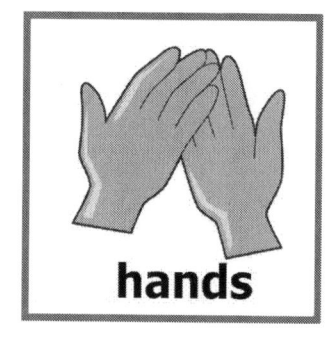

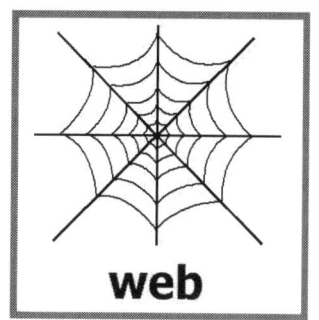

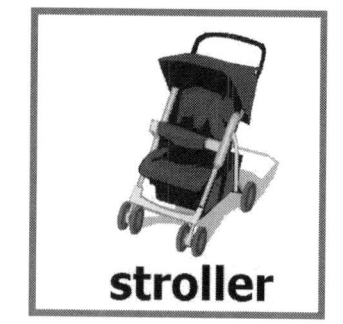

airplane

tree

tiger

hands

web

stroller

Joggin' Your Noggin
Word Pairs
Board F6

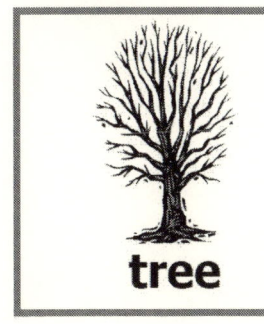

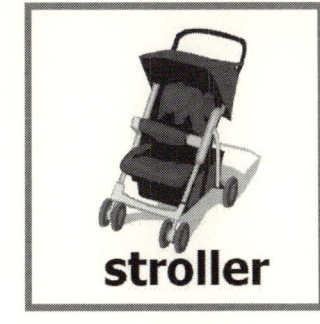

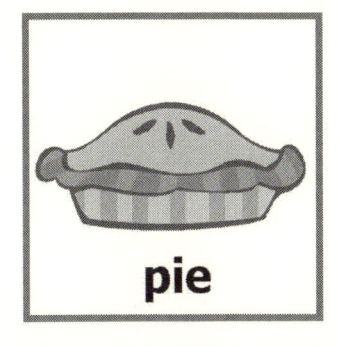

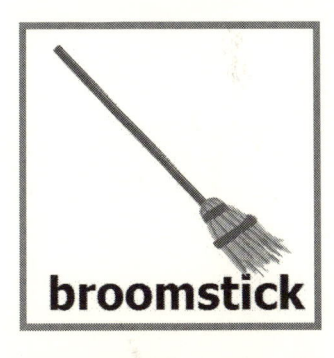

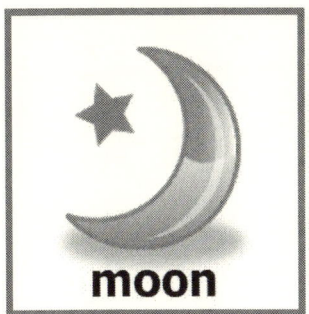

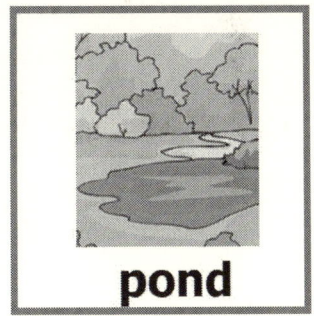

tree	stroller
pie	broomstick
moon	pond

Made in the USA
Coppell, TX
14 April 2022